*ALL THE VERY
BEST IN HEALTH
AND FITNESS.*

Get
Lean
and
Healthy

Todd T. Matthews, BA, RHN, RNCP, CSCS

This book is not intended to diagnose, treat, prevent, or cure any disease. Before you start any nutritional plan, consult with a doctor who is familiar with your health history.

Contents

Chapter 1: Introduction

A Call to Action

You are about to begin the greatest weight loss program ever developed. This program is the best because it makes no compromises on your health and encourages the consumption of healthy fruit, vegetables, and quality protein. Clients have lost as much as 12 pounds in the first week, although losing 3 to 8 pounds in the first week is more typical. After the first week, you can expect an incredible 1 to 3 pound weight loss every week! This system is the culmination of the best ideas from scientific research as well as my own experience -- from more than 10 years helping people lose weight.

Now is the time for a change. Now is the time for you to get the lean and healthy body you deserve.

Do you feel self conscious because of your weight? Do you wear a one piece bathing suit instead of a bikini? Do you swim with a T-shirt on to cover up your body, not to protect you from the sun? Does walking up a set of stairs make you out of breath because you're carrying extra weight? Do your joints hurt doing everyday activities? Do you feel just slightly overweight but are struggling to lose the last few pounds? Life is too short for such rubbish! You deserve a lean and sexy body that is charged with vibrant health. This body you have is your body for life; it should be one you're proud of.

Diets Don't Work

This is not a diet because diets don't work. Diets can help you lose weight initially, but, unless you commit to a new way of eating for life, you'll eventually gain all the weight back. If you are overweight, the way you eat is the biggest culprit of what has made you overweight. I know some of you are thinking that it is a lack of exercise in your lifestyle that has made you gain fat; not true. If you eat properly, you can go through long periods of inactivity without gaining weight. To get lean fast, just follow this system, but to stay lean, you must follow the Stay Lean Maintenance Phase as well. This journey is going to make a permanent change in your lifestyle, one that you must be ready to adopt for life. If you ever go back to your old way of eating, you will return to being overweight.

Why the Get Lean and Healthy System was Developed

After a few years as a personal trainer, I realized exercise alone does not serve as the most efficient way to lose weight. Clients, adhering to my exercise programs, were weight training three times a week and doing up to four hours of cardiovascular exercise a week. Yet, some of them were not losing weight! How was this possible? They were burning about 500 calories per workout, which averages to about 3500 calories a week. As there are 3500 calories in a single pound of fat, that should be enough to drop 1 pound in a week. So, what exactly was the problem here?

As it turns out, the problem was improper eating habits.

Here's how it works. Somewhere between 500 and 600 calories is perhaps the most energy the average sized person can burn from a one hour session of vigorous weight or cardiovascular training. But, an ice cream cone with a single scoop also contains as much as 500 to 600 calories. So, while in one hour you can burn off around 500 calories, you can also eat 500 calories in about 10 minutes. It's a myth that you can exercise hard, eat anything you want, and have a lean body.

I soon realized that I needed to add a nutritional component to my training programs for my clients. Over the years, I have experimented with many diets, using myself and my clients as test subjects. The traditional weight loss diets on the market were too complicated, unhealthy, or ineffective, for one reason or another. And, after many years of academic study using the best and latest scientific research as well as finding out what works for my clients, I've discovered the ultimate diet. It works for everybody. Do you have a slow metabolism? This system will work for you. Have you always been overweight? This system will work for you. Have you been unsuccessful on a million other diets? This system will work for you. Using this system, you will feel healthy and reach your weight loss goals, but you must stick to the program.

The Get Lean and Healthy style of eating allows you to stay lean when you're not able to exercise. At some point in your life, you may be forced to stop exercising for a period of time. You may have to recover from an injury or finish a thesis. A few weeks or months may go by where you can't workout. You need to know your system of eating will not make your weight creep back toward obesity if you can't exercise.

So, creating a diet centered upon optimal health was crucial for me. This system promotes good health and will also help you lose weight. The Get Lean and Healthy system is the healthiest dieting system on the planet and the very best tool for weight loss.

Following the GLH program with 100% of your commitment and dedication is essential. Little variations in the program can throw off the delicate balance, leading to little or no progress. As little as one muffin and one half of a bagel eaten during the course of a week can halt your progress for that entire week. You also can't miss meals. The meals and snacks on the program are essential parts of the process. Skipping meals is not a part of the system and should be avoided. Eat every three hours. If you don't eat enough, you'll slow down your metabolism, leading to a halt in your daily progress. This system is all about balance. If you follow it, it will work.

The Secret to Weight Loss 70-25-5

The secret to permanent weight loss is the 70-25-5 rule. Regarding weight loss, diet is 70% of the battle, exercise is 25%, and supplements are 5%. The fitness magazines are stuffed with ads from supplement manufacturers trying to make you believe supplements are your key to weight loss. Supplements can help give you a slight edge, but what you eat is really what will make or break you. Exercise is far more important than supplements, but nothing is as important as the food you actually put into your body. Exercise helps, of course, but until you address your diet, you won't see much progress toward your healthy weight goals.

Chapter 2: Why the System Works

Why the Get Lean and Healthy system works so well

Simply and briefly stated:

1.	Portion control leads to fewer overall calories ingested.

2.	This system demands an adequate consumption of fat, fiber, and protein, along with decreased consumption of high glycemic index carbohydrates. Eating this way stabilizes blood sugar levels, reducing the fat storing effects of the hormone insulin and increasing the fat burning effects of the hormone glucagon – all this leads to rapid, healthy weight loss.

3.	GLH also weans you from your addiction to sweet tasting foods and large portions of starchy foods. Why is this important? It is the high consumption of sugary and starchy foods that causes fat gain. These foods literally trigger insulin to store fat and to keep piling on the pounds!

Stay with me and all of this will be explained in further detail.

Some carbohydrate foods are dense with starch or high in sugar. How does bread, pasta, or sweets trigger the body to store fat? Starchy carbohydrates, flour products, and sugary foods raise blood sugar quickly. Elevated blood sugar must be immediately lowered and having very high blood sugar levels is quite dangerous. Insulin lowers blood sugar by storing the sugar – pumping it into the cells – which makes you fatter. Now, you do need a certain amount of insulin to survive, but very high levels lead to metabolic syndrome diseases such as heart disease, type II diabetes, high blood pressure, and a poor cholesterol ratio.

So, how can this be prevented?

A. Eat smaller portions of carbohydrates at each meal.
B. Eat carbohydrates in combination with FAT, FIBER, and/or PROTEIN.
C. Limit high starch and sugar foods.

Fiber, protein, and fat all slow down your digestion process and lets the sugar from carbohydrates trickle into the blood stream more slowly. This gives you a steady stream of energy and lets your body burn more fat.

Glucagon, a fat burning hormone secreted from the pancreas, is elevated by the increased protein consumed and the lowered, or rather, normal blood sugar levels present in your system. Glucagon burns fat.

Insulin, a storage hormone, is reduced, therefore lessening excess sugar storage and, ultimately, fat.

The Science of Weight Loss

If we look at the science of weight loss, there are two primary factors that contribute to losing weight.

The Calorie Factor

First, there is the calorie factor. If you eat more calories than you burn, you will gain weight. On the other hand, if you burn more calories than you consume, you will lose weight. Therefore, less food consumption and more exercise will obviously help with weight loss.

The Hormone Factor

Hormones are powerful metabolic messengers directing the body to behave in certain ways. Hormones are related to stress, gender, energy production, sleep, and many other functions and processes in the body.

The hormone insulin forces the body to store fat and the hormone glucagon directs the body to burn fat.

If we can control these hormones, then, ultimately, we can control the process of getting lean. Good news; these hormones can be influenced by the foods we eat.

If we look at a day long graph of blood sugar (figure A) we can see how fat burning hormones are influenced by foods.

The graph shows high, low, and normal blood sugar levels. The dotted line represents the blood sugar of a person consuming the Standard American Diet. The solid line represents the blood sugar of a person on the Get Lean and Healthy system.

How Blood Sugar Levels Effect Weight Gain and Weight Loss

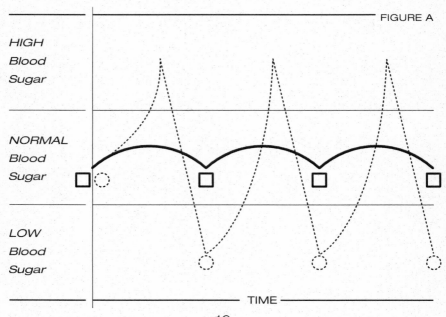

FIGURE A

....
STANDARD NORTH AMERICAN DIET
- Increased insulin.
- Increased body fat.
- Instable blood sugar reduces ones ability to perform and concentrate.

STANDARD NORTH AMERICAN MEAL

─────────────
GET LEAN AND HEALTHY DIET
- Increased glucagon.
- Decreased body fat.
- Stable blood sugar for increased athletic performance and concentration.

☐ *GET LEAN AND HEALTHY MEAL*

A person on the Standard American Diet (SAD) will be a fat storage machine. Blood sugar after a SAD meal is elevated rapidly to a very high level. This can be seen on the first upward slope of the dotted line. Insulin is secreted at the peak, when blood sugar levels get too high and turn the excess blood sugar into fat. The fat storage of the excess blood sugar can be seen as the steep downward slope of the dotted line. I call this the storage slope. The storage slope must be avoided if you want to stay lean for life.

For the person on the GLH system, represented by the solid line, blood sugar levels never get too high or too low. This ensures insulin, which is always present in the body, never gets high enough to force the body to become a fat storage machine. Insulin, our fat storage hormone, is reduced. Glucagon, our fat burning hormone, is increased.

Let's look at the dietary habits of a person on the Standard American Diet. The person on the SAD wakes up and gets ready for work. On the way to work, this person goes though a drive-through, picking up a low fat muffin and a large orange juice for breakfast. Many would think this is a healthy breakfast; however, as you will soon see, this breakfast will make you fat, especially if consumed on any sort of regular basis.

Fruit juice is simply the water, sugar, and vitamins extracted from fruit.

So, what's wrong with that? Two things: first, the provided carbohydrate/sugar quantity is too high and, second, there is no fiber. It is the fiber in the original fruit that slows the uptake of carbohydrates/sugar from the orange. Never drink juice. Always eat whole fruit. The processing of the fruit itself into juice removes the fiber that your body so desperately needs to keep blood sugar stable. (The same process happens, of course, when you drink cola, and by cola, we mean any soda, soft drink, or pop.)

Get an orange, cut it in half, and squeeze both halves into a glass. How much juice did you get? Is there one inch in the bottom of the glass? Maybe there is, but only if the orange being juiced was large to begin with. It takes eight, ten, maybe twelve oranges to fill a large glass with juice. Imagine that – the juice, or the sugar, of twelve oranges. This is way too much sugar for the body to process. This much sugar, eaten alone, rapidly raises the body's blood sugar. To prevent blood sugar from getting dangerously high, insulin stores the excess blood sugar as fat.

Now, for the second part of our breakfast. A low-fat muffin also has a great deal of carbohydrates. Most muffins are made with enriched white flour. White flour starts as whole grain flour, but, after processing, ends up with all of the healthy fiber removed. Most store bought or commercial bran muffins are surprisingly low in fiber. Muffins are also low in protein. Protein slows down the digestion of carbohydrates, leading to stable blood sugar and, therefore, less fat storage. This muffin is also low-fat. Fat, it should be remembered, can be a good thing. Fat slows down the digestion process, leading to a more stable blood sugar level and less fat storage. So, a low fat muffin is high in carbohydrates, but low on the basic elements (fat, fiber, protein) which help prevent carbohydrates from making you fat.

Between the sugar of up to twelve oranges in the juice and a high load of carbohydrates in the low-fat muffin, eating this for breakfast will make you fat.

GLH, with the help of fat, fiber, and protein, and, therefore, the hormone glucagon, forces the body to lose fat. It also takes into account portion control via the palm rule, which helps limit calorie intake (although calories are not proportioned to be so low that you're hungry). This leads to optimum fat loss.

Another hormone relating to body fat is leptin. Leptin is a hormone circulating at levels proportionate to body fat. The higher the leptin levels are, the higher the body fat percentage will be. Studies show that people who eat a primitive/natural diet have far lower leptin levels than people eating a modern diet of refined and processed foods.

In one study of two tribes in Tanzania, one tribe ate a vegetarian diet while the other ate a diet adding a high intake of fish. The tribes lived identical lifestyles and their nutrition was similar, except for the inclusion of fish in the one tribe's diet. The fish tribe had 25% lower levels of leptin. Eating fish and/or taking fish oil supplements helps reduce leptin levels and, thus, body-fat.

Another way to lower leptin levels is with sleep. Leptin levels are down-regulated by melatonin, a hormone released at night in association with sleep. More sleep or better quality sleep equals lower leptin and lower body-fat. An adequate amount of high quality sleep is also great for your overall health.

Therefore, the amount of fat you burn is increased mainly by four things: increased exercise, increased protein consumption, careful carbohydrate consumption, and increased fish oil consumption. GLH will have you doing all of these. As per the GLH rules, you must eat a palm size serving of protein with every meal, eliminate refined carbohydrates, and exercise at least 30 minutes a day.

Get Lean and Healthy is the Healthiest Diet on the Planet

Why is GLH the healthiest diet ever?

1. On this program you'll be eating vegetables more than anything else. Vegetables are higher in antioxidants (as well as many other vitamins and minerals) than any other food group.

2. There are no artificial sweeteners on the program. Although this is not 100% agreed upon, many researchers say that, at the very least, artificial sweeteners are mild toxins.

3. The system has adequate protein to rebuild muscles, hormones, and other tissues. There is also enough protein at meals to make the body circulate more glucagon. Remember, glucagon is a potent fat burning hormone.

4. There is a balanced source of essential fats. All healthy types of fats are consumed on this program, including monounsaturated fats from olive oil, saturated fats (in moderation) from lean meats, and polyunsaturated fats from nuts, fish oil, and seafood.

5. No trans-fats. Trans-fats are hydrogenated fats and should be treated like poison to the body. They are used in many packaged foods, baked goods, and cookies. French fries and other deep fried fast foods, like fish burgers and fried chicken, are usually fried in trans-fats.

6. No nitrates. Nitrates are the carcinogenic (cancer causing) preservatives added to cold-meats/processed meats. Do not eat nitrates... Ever.

Chapter 3: Rapid Weight Loss

This healthy weight loss plan focuses on natural food the human body performs best on. This protocol emphasizes health-promoting fruits and vegetables, adequate protein, and essential fatty acids. By following the rules below, you will lose between 3-12 pounds the first week and 1-3 pounds every week after until you reach your ideal weight.

Why does this program work? First, the diet increases fat burning hormones in the body. Second, it decreases fat storage hormones in the body. Third, it decreases overall calories to help you lose weight. Additionally, it is high enough in calories to keep your metabolism up. It is also not a low carbohydrate diet. This is a low refined carbohydrate diet, which is very healthy.

The Get Lean and Healthy Program Rules:

1. The Palm Rule
Each meal consists of a palm sized portion of protein eaten with unlimited greens and fibrous vegetables. A fist sized portion of high fiber fruit between meals is encouraged as a snack.

2. The Three Hour Rule
Never go more than 3 hours between meals.

3. The Water Rule
Drink 1L of water for every 50 pounds of bodyweight per day.

4. The Exercise Rule

Exercise vigorously for at least 30 minutes every day.

5. The Natural Food Rule

Whenever possible, eat natural, whole, and preferably organic foods.

Follow these simple rules and you'll have the body you've always wanted in no time.

1. The Palm Rule

At every meal, consume a palm sized portion of quality protein with an unlimited amount of fibrous vegetables

Look at your palm. Now, without including your fingers or your thumb, the mass of your palm is the protein portion you should eat at each meal. (As well as being the portion size of starchy carbohydrates you can consume during the maintenance phase.) Along with your protein, you can eat unlimited amounts of salad and fibrous vegetables.

Rapid Weight Loss Meal

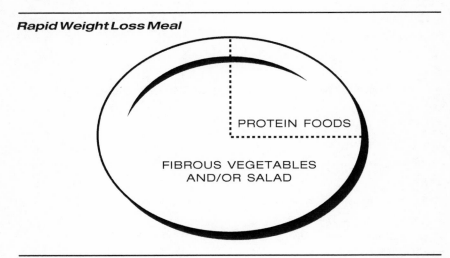

PROTEIN FOODS

FIBROUS VEGETABLES
AND/OR SALAD

A little oil and vinegar dressing is acceptable. Try to make your own dressings and use high quality oils. Most store bought dressing is high in sugar, salt, and preservatives, so you should avoid them.

Example of a healthy Salad Dressing:

A. Extra virgin olive oil - 1tbsp (Or any expeller pressed, cold pressed or extra virgin oil - flax oil would be fantastic)

B. Vinegar - 1 tbsp (Balsamic vinegar, red wine vinegar, lime juice, or lemon juice)

C. Dijon Mustard (optional; to taste)

D. Spices, pepper, herbs (to taste)

E. Water - 1 tbsp (Adding water to dressings cuts down on the dryness of a salad without adding calories. Look at the ingredient list of many low calorie dressings and you will find extra water has been added when compared to their full calorie dressing counterparts.)

For snacks, you should have a fist-sized portion (or less) of high fiber fruit. The high fiber fruit stabilizes your blood sugar, which allows your body to burn fat. Examples of high fiber fruit are discussed later in this chapter.

The palm rule allows you to determine the portion of protein you should be eating at each meal. This helps you manage portions to keep calories relatively low and your blood sugar stable. For rapid healthy weight loss, it is crucial to keep your blood sugar stable to avoid the fat storage effects of the insulin hormone. Fiber, protein, and fat all slow the digestion of carbohydrates. The slowdown of the digestion of carbohydrates leads to stable blood sugar, because the carbohydrates slowly enter the blood stream instead of flooding it.

GLH meals must contain protein and fiber rich vegetables. Snacks must contain high fiber fruit. This style of eating reduces the fat storage effects of insulin that carbohydrates can trigger. Fat, fiber, and protein are your friends in the weight loss game. They all help slow the digestion of carbohydrates and lead to stable blood sugar levels. GLH will give you lots of energy as well as fat and weight loss.

It is important that you eat enough protein. Studies show a diet higher in protein consumption results in a sustained reduction in appetite. Protein makes you feel full and keeps you satisfied longer than carbohydrates. Protein, therefore, leads to less consumption, leading to greater weight loss. Studies also show that protein consumption supports lean body mass, which preserves metabolism during weight loss. Muscle weight must be maintained during weight loss as muscle burns many calories even at rest. Muscle is fat burning tissue; you don't want to lose an ounce of it. As we age, we tend to lose muscle starting at about age 35. The battle is to keep as much muscle as possible.

2. Three Hour Rule

Never go more than three hours without eating

It is optimal to eat 5 to 6 small meals or snacks per day at 2 to 3 hour intervals. This gives your body tissues a constant supply of nutrients and energy. These regular smaller feedings lessen the risk of fat storage from the excess calories gained from having one large meal.

3. The Water Rule

1 liter (4 cups) per 50 pounds of bodyweight per day

For example, a 150-pound person should drink 3 liters (12 cups) of water per day. Water is needed for many reactions in the body. It is necessary for the breakdown of stored body-fat. This breakdown of fat is called a hydrolysis reaction. Fat may be broken down more slowly in someone who is dehydrated. Water can also be an appetite suppressant, because many people who over eat are really just thirsty. Some people improperly interpret signals from their body and think they are hungry when they are really thirsty.

It would be ideal to drink only water. However, on this program, you can have other calorie free/low calorie drinks in moderation, such as coffee, tea, herbal tea, and water with fresh lemon. If drinking tea and/or coffee, keep it unsweetened. Reduce coffee consumption as it can adversely affect blood sugar, therefore, slowing weight loss in some people. (Elimination of coffee should be a long term goal; however, with all of the dietary changes you are making, giving up caffeine or coffee as well can be too much for some people.)

Soft drinks are not acceptable in any phase of the GLH. Soft drinks are detrimental to your health due to additives, color, artificial sweeteners, and sugar. The average cola has 14 teaspoons of sugar -- try that in your tea and see how it tastes. The sugar in cola will kill your chances of weight loss.

Juice can also make you gain weight because of its concentrated sugar levels. It takes several fruits to make an 8-12oz glass of juice -- more whole fruits than you would ever eat at one sitting. Stay away from juice and, instead, eat whole fruits to keep your body lean.

Ice tea and fruit flavored beverages are just as bad as soft drinks. Again, water is your best choice.

Alcohol is not permitted on GLH. It has too many calories and too few vitamins, minerals, and antioxidants. A 12oz bottle of beer has 140-150 calories; even light beer has between 100-120 calories. A glass of wine has 110-130 calories and a 1.5oz shot of liquor has 100-150 calories. A Martini has 400 calories, a rum and cola 240, and a vodka and cranberry has 250.

If you're drinking 2 alcoholic beverages a day and stop, you will lose 2 pounds a month. (This assumes that you keep your food intake and exercise levels consistent.)

There is another reason besides adding empty calories not to drink alcohol: Alcohol is a drug which the liver must detoxify out of the blood stream. The liver, which detoxifies the body, also breaks down fats in the body. If the liver is not functioning optimally, fat loss may be slower due to inefficient breakdown of fats. Do not drink alcohol on the rapid weight loss phase for optimal fat loss. Drink moderately during the maintenance phase to stay lean.

4. The Exercise Rule

Exercise for at least 30 minutes Every Day

Any exercise and or vigorous activity burns calories and leads to weight loss. Exercise does not need to be structured exercise in a gym or fitness center. Walking, biking, swimming, or even dancing counts as exercise. Do any activity that elevates your heart rate and puts a demand on your muscles.

If you can't exercise everyday, you should try to attain an average of 3.5 hours of exercise per week. A little over an hour for three days a week works well for many people.

The best form of exercise for weight loss is resistance training or strength training. This may be a shock to you, as it is a shock to most people. Weight training is great for weight loss because it speeds up the metabolism for up to 48 hours after the session leading to the greatest fat loss. However, if not performed properly, weight training can lead to muscle imbalances and even injuries. Consult with a certified fitness professional.

The program works even if you don't exercise at all. But, you won't look as good or feel as good if you don't exercise. The healthy, athletic look is only achieved by a combination of diet and exercise.

Do not increase your current amount of physical activity before assessing your ability to do so by filling out a Par-Q and/or getting clearance from your doctor.

5. Natural Food Rule

Eat only foods you could hunt and gather

The human body evolved to thrive on a diet based on sourcing food through hunting and gathering. There were no refined foods in the diet that our bodies were designed to eat. Live this mantra: Eat only foods you could hunt and gather. Please note, however, that there are a few notable exceptions of super-foods you could not hunt or gather. Yogurt, for instance, is a super food.

Fruits, meats, poultry, seafood, vegetables, seeds, and nuts must be the bulk of your diet. Packaged foods, cured meats, flour products, and refined sugar containing products have no place in a healthy diet.

Wait, I know what you're thinking. Why no flour products? Our bodies simply haven't evolved to be able to deal with the increased blood sugar spike which occurs when we consume flour products like breads, muffins, cakes, donuts, and pastries. Human evolution happened slowly over about two million years. The consumption of grains and flour products is still relatively new. Only during the last ten thousand years have these agricultural foods become a big part of our diet. Our hunt and gather ancestors lived on a diet of fresh fruits, vegetables, fish, and game. Flour products are high on the glycemic index and, therefore, tend to spike blood sugar and trigger our fat storage hormones. If you want to be lean, eat like a caveman or cavewoman.

Refined sugar products do an even better job of spiking blood sugar and cause our bodies to become fat storage machines. To lose weight:

Never eat any refined sugar or any flour products

- Bread is cake
- Muffins are cake

It's the truth!
Replace all flour products with antioxidant rich fruits and vegetables.

I know what you're thinking, "But, I love my muffin in the morning!" Well... Do you love your thighs? Do you love your bottom? Do you love your cellulite? Do you love your spare tire? Do you love your belly? If the food you love is making you miserable, then you're being foolish. Sugar and flour products will make you gain weight. Remember the following:

Sweet Taste = Fat Body.   Starchy and Satisfying = Fat Body

People say, "Wow, this is a great cake. Delicious." They should be saying, "This cake will put me at risk for diabetes, heart disease, certain cancers, and will make me overweight, thereby putting unnec-essary strain on my joints and leading to possible joint replacement in the future. This cake will make me fat, so I will look awful in a bathing suit". Harsh, but, for some, this reality check is necessary. A lifestyle change must happen for you to lose weight permanently. Admitting the truth is necessary for getting your weight down and keeping it off.

Your colon is one more reason to reduce your consumption of flour products. How do you teach young children to make glue? Mix flour and water. This is not a good recipe for having regular bowel movements. The human body evolved to need a large amount of fiber to function optimally. Reducing your intake of pasta, bread, and baked goods will help you lose weight and feel healthier, but it will also make your colon happier. Remember, flour products tend to be higher in starch and also lower in vitamins, minerals, and fiber than are fruits and vegetables.

Watch out for hidden sugars in sauces and spreads like Ketchup, BBQ sauce, peanut butter, jam, teriyaki sauce, and plum sauce. Most sauces are loaded with sugar -- because it's cheap. Check ingredients on product labels for sugar in the form of cane sugar, raw sugar, fructose, maltose, dextrose, sucrose, high fructose corn syrup, corn syrup, etc. (Anything with –ose at the end is a type of sugar.) All of the above ingredients are just other names for sugar. A high consumption of refined sugars eventually causes weight gain through the power of insulin. Not to mention, there are lots of other ways to season your food. Try using dry herbs and spices, fresh herbs, garlic, and sauces and salsas containing no sugar. Always check the labels of foods you buy and go organic whenever possible.

Refined sugars deplete vitamins. Every time you ingest a food, it needs to be broken down fully, assimilated by the body, and then built back up into structured and/or stored energy for the body. Vitamins are catalysts; they assist in the processing of these components of food. Fruits and vegetables contain an abundance of vitamins. When you eat fruits or vegetables, you get vitamins to assist in the processing of food components. Refined sugar is nothing but pure carbohydrates, containing no vitamins and no minerals. There are no vitamins and minerals to help process the sugar, and no vitamins and minerals to help with other processes in the body. Your body must supply vitamins to process the sugar you have eaten; so, eating sugar depletes the body of vitamins.

Many food products contain artificial ingredients, artificial flavors, artificial sweeteners, additives, and preservatives. These substances have no place in a healthy diet. Eat nutritious natural foods.

Healthy bodies look good from the inside out.

On the GLH program, artificial sweeteners must not be consumed. Many studies suggest artificial sweeteners are unhealthy and poisonous to our bodies. Not all studies show danger in consuming these products; however, the consumption of these relatively new substances to your system makes you a guinea pig. I'll stick with fresh fruit to get my sweet fix, thanks!

More importantly, the ingestion of these artificial sweeteners does not wean you from the addiction to very sweet tasting foods. With a diet high in artificial sugar, you may lose weight, but you won't keep it off because, at the end of the program, you'll still crave sweet, sugary foods. After a couple of weeks on the Get Lean and Healthy program, very sweet foods will taste too sweet and cravings for them will all but disappear.

Try to consume more organic foods. Organic foods are pesticide free. Sounds great, but why is that a good thing? Pesticides kill bugs by wiping out the bug's neurological system. The neurological system includes the brain, spinal cord, and other nerves. So, pesticides are, at the very least, mildly toxic to the brain of humans. Organic foods cost more, but it's a good place to spend your money. Buying certified organic foods is better than spending money on supplements. (Buying organic foods is even better than buying the supplements recommended in this book.) Really, there is nothing special about organic foods. They're just food – just as nature intended. Until about 50 years ago, organic was the only choice.

The Program Outline

In a nutshell, here's the program: Eat 5-6 times per day; 3 meals and 2-3 snacks. Eat using the following template below.

Rapid Weight Loss Phase Outline (1000-1800Kcal)

Meal 1   Protein – palm sized portion
Fruit – palm sized portion
Yogurt – palm sized portion

or

Nutrition Shake (recipe is at the end of this chapter)

Snack   Fruit – fist sized portion

Meal 2   Protein – palm sized portion
Vegetables – unlimited

Snack   Fruit – fist sized portion

Meal 3   Protein – palm sized portion
Vegetables – unlimited

*If you're hungry, raw vegetables can be consumed between meals.

Examples of Protein Sources:

Fish, seafood, chicken, tofu, lean pork, lean beef, lamb, eggs, turkey, bison, venison, ostrich, and whey protein isolate.
(Avoid processed and cured deli meats, bacon, and ham.)

Examples of Non-starchy/High fiber/Low GI Vegetables:

Green/red/orange/yellow sweet peppers, cucumber, zucchini, kale, sprouts, leeks, artichokes, spinach, broccoli, brussel sprouts, tomatoes, cabbage, chard, collards, asparagus, cabbage, cauliflower, lettuce, any mixed greens, onions, and mushrooms. (Avoid potatoes, carrots, and other starchy tubers during the rapid weight loss period.)

Beans (legumes) are not on the GLH Rapid Weight Loss Phase due to their high carbohydrate content. However, legumes in their pods (green beans, snow peas) should be treated like vegetables and are, therefore, perfect for the rapid weight loss phase. The pod supplies a lot of fiber, lowering the ratio of carbohydrate to fiber and lowering the foods ranking on the glycemic index. (Legumes out of their pods can be eaten during maintenance as long as the portion does not exceed palm size. The legumes must also be eaten with a palm sized portion of protein.)

Bean sprouts can also be eaten on the Rapid Weight Loss phase. Sprouting a legume makes the legume more like a vegetable. As a sprouted legume begins to turn into a plant, the amount of starch is reduced and lowers the bean's rating on the glycemic index. For this system, consider bean sprouts to be vegetables not legumes and eat as much as you want. (Sprouting beans also makes them healthier. I will share why later.)

When I say you should eat high fiber vegetables in unlimited quantities, I mean that you should eat a lot of vegetables. You should eat 2-5 pounds of vegetables each and every day. Eat as much high fiber vegetables as all of the other food you're eating combined. Vegetables are extremely healthy because of their high fiber content and antioxidant levels.

Examples of Fruit Portions:

1 apple, 1 pear, 1 peach, 1 orange, 2 kiwis, 2 plums, 6 strawberries, ½ grapefruit, ¼ honeydew melon, ¼ cantaloupe melon, 1 cup berries, or 1 cup grapes.
(Avoid bananas during the rapid weight loss phase.)

Starchy Carbohydrate Sources:

There are **NO starchy carbohydrates**, such as grains (all baked products), potatoes, rice, pasta, or legumes, on the rapid weight loss phase. These foods will be added back into your diet during the maintenance phase.

Dairy Products:

Dairy products are both a protein and a carbohydrate based food; about a 60:40 ratio of carbohydrate to protein. (Fat content varies; cream has 18% milk fat and skim milk has none.)

Plain yogurt should be eaten almost daily. I would define yogurt as a super food. Yogurt contains acidophilus, a very healthy bacteria that is excellent for your digestive system. Some yogurts contain other types of similar healthy bacteria as well. This bacteria is natural and is a healthy part of your colon, and can lead to better overall health.

Exactly why acidophilus is so healthy is outside of the scope of this book; for now just eat it and reap the health benefits.

Other dairy products are not recommended as they are hard to digest. (The lactose in yogurt is pre-digested by the bacteria culture.)

Top Foods for a Healthy Body

Below is a list of the top foods for optimal health.
Many of these foods can help prevent certain diseases. These foods contain antioxidants, minerals, essential fats, and bioflavonoids. These important nutrients can help prevent ailments like diabetes, heart disease, and certain cancers. The food you decide to eat can have great effects on your health.

Eating more of the suggested foods below not only makes you feel great, but gives you more energy.

Suggested Protein Foods

These are the best protein foods to eat as based on the following: associated fat quality, protein quality, digestibility, vitamins, and minerals. Most of these protein sources are also widely available; this is taken into account as well.

Fish and Seafood
- Cod
- Halibut
- Herring (*lower contamination)
- Salmon
- Sardines (*lower contamination)
- Scallops
- Shrimp
- Snapper
- Tuna

Some wild and most farmed fish are contaminated with toxins and mercury. This is a concern as fish without toxins are such a healthy food. To reduce the amount of toxins you take in when selecting fish, remember the following:

1. Larger fish are more contaminated than smaller fish. Therefore sardines and herring may be the best choices for fish intake.

2. The higher on the food-chain fish are, the higher the contamination levels.

3. Farmed fish are more contaminated than wild caught fish.

All fish are somewhat contaminated with mercury, a potent neurotoxin. Because of the mercury contamination, current research suggests limiting fish intake to two times a month, for adults, and entirely eliminating fish intake for pregnant mothers, lactating mothers, and infants. However, the Omega 3 fatty acids in fish are healthy for the heart and brain, so pharmaceutical grade or contaminant-free fish oil should be taken daily by almost everyone. The EPA and DHA in fish oil have also been shown to accelerate fat loss in those who consume it. EPA (eicosapentanoic acid) and DHA (docosahexanoic acid) are Omega 3 fatty acids that contribute to brain health and can reduce the risk of cardiovascular disease.

Poultry, Eggs, Dairy and Meat
- Lean Beef
- Bison
- Chicken
- Cottage Cheese
- Eggs
- Lamb
- Ostrich
- Turkey
- Venison
- Whey Protein Isolate

Mixed Protein and Carbohydrate Foods (40:60 Ratio)
- Yogurt

Suggested Carbohydrate Foods

These carbohydrate foods are selected because of their relatively high fiber content (in particular, soluble fiber) and low glycemic index value as well as vitamin, mineral, and antioxidant levels.

High Fiber Vegetables

- Asparagus
- Avocado
- Bell peppers
- Broccoli
- Brussels sprouts
- Cabbage
- Cauliflower
- Celery
- Collard greens
- Cucumber
- Eggplant
- Fennel bulb
- Garlic
- Green beans
- Kale
- Leeks
- Mushrooms
- Mustard greens
- Olives
- Onions
- Parsley
- Romaine lettuce
- Sea Vegetables
- Spinach
- Squash (any type)
- Swiss chard
- Tomato
- Turnip greens

High Fiber Fruit

(During the rapid weight loss stage, only eat fresh fruits; avoid dried fruits.)

- Apple
- Apricot
- Blueberries
- Cranberries
- Grapefruit
- Grapes
- Kiwi fruit
- Lemons
- Limes
- Melon (any)
- Orange
- Papaya
- Pear
- Pineapple
- Plums
- Raspberries
- Strawberries

Suggested Healthy Fat and Oil Based Foods

(Consume in moderation. These foods are high in calories.)

- Almonds
- Avocado
- Brazil Nuts
- Cashews
- Flax Seeds / Flax Oil (do not cook)*
- Olive Oil, Extra Virgin
- Pumpkin Seeds
- Sesame Seeds / Oil (do not cook)*
- Sunflower Seeds / Oil (do not cook)*
- Walnuts

(*Heating these oils denatures them)

Example Menu:
Rapid Weight Loss Phase

Menu A

Meal 1   Nutrition Shake (with frozen berries)

Snack   1 Apple

Meal 2   Chicken Caesar Salad (1 whole chicken breast)
Whole raw red pepper
½ cucumber

Snack   2 plums

Meal 3   Palm sized lean steak
Grilled Sliced Zucchini (2-3 whole)
Large Greek Salad

Menu B

Meal 1   2 boiled eggs
1 cup fresh strawberries with 1 cup plain yogurt

Snack   1 Pear

Meal 2   Lean turkey Sausage (2)
   – must be nitrate and preservative free
2 cups of steamed broccoli
1 cup of raw cauliflower

Snack   2 Kiwi fruit (Gooseberry fruit)

Meal 3   Wild salmon steak or filet – palm size
Grilled Asparagus (10-15)
Grilled Portobello Mushrooms (2-3)
Mixed baby greens with olive oil, red wine vinegar and
Dijon mustard

Variety Is a Must

Eat a wide variety of different foods. Your diet will only be optimum if you eat a variety of foods as each food is high in some nutrients but deficient in others. Apples are very high in the soluble fiber pectin, which is excellent as it is very cleansing on the digestive system. Apples are lower in vitamins and antioxidants than other fruits, such as melon and berries which do not have quite as much fiber. As a rule, try to never eat the same food two days in a row; in other words, try to go 48 hours before consuming the same food again.

Eating more of the suggested foods not only makes you feel great, but gives you more energy.

Milk

Why is there no milk on the GLH system? There are two main reasons. First, milk is a food you drink; a fairly complete food. It has protein, carbohydrates, fats, vitamins, and minerals. (Milk contains no fiber, however.) Milk is a dense source of liquid calories. For someone trying to lose weight, it is an extra source of calories but it is not as satisfying as eating solid food. For this reason, it is can be an excellent food for someone trying to gain weight (if they can digest it) and a bad food for someone trying to lose weight.

Milk also has another deficiency. It is not digested well by many people. Much of the human population is lactose intolerant, so they can't drink milk without supplemental lactose enzymes. This is not a problem with yogurt; lactose intolerant individuals can eat yogurt (with live bacteria culture) as the bacteria has broken down the lactose.

The Get Lean Weekly Weight Loss Recorder: Example

On the Get Lean and Healthy system, you will weigh yourself once a week. Pick a day, Monday, Tuesday, or whatever day you most prefer, and stick with it for the duration of the program. For each weigh-in, weigh yourself at the same time of day and wear similar clothing. Try to use the same scale for accuracy, if possible. Also, keep in mind that weighing yourself in the morning gives the most accurate measurement.

Some people find they are more motivated if they get on the scale every day. This may tend to stop people from slipping backward. The only problem with is that after the first week, you'll only be losing 1-3 pounds a week and that may not show up as a daily change.

Below is an actual case study. As you can see, Bill lost a lot of weight in the first week and, then, the weight loss slowed down quite a bit. This is typical; however, this case is a bit extreme. Bill was falling off the program by week 5 when he cheated (ribs, dessert, and 2 beers). Bill ate one large meal off of the system and his weight loss stopped dead in its tracks.

	Date	**Weight**
Week 1	*May 20*	238
Week 2	*May 27*	227.5
Week 3	*June 3*	226.5
Week 4	*June 10*	224.5
Week 5	*June 17*	222
Week 6	*June 24*	222
Week 7	*July 1*	218.5
Week 8	*July 7*	214.5
Week 9	*July 14*	213.5
Week 10	*July 21*	212

Follow the program 100% of the time. Adherence to the program 95% of the time will just not do. If you don't follow the program 100%, you may lose weight at a snails pace or you may not lose weight at all. You could actually gain weight.

Remember this phase is temporary. You do not have to eat this way forever; just until you lose all the weight you want to. Then, you can start the maintenance phase.

Nutrition Shakes!

Short on time? In a rush? Try this handy meal replacement.

Blend and enjoy the following ingredients:

Delicious Berry Recipe:

Water	125ml/ 0.5cup
Yogurt (plain /unsweetened)	250g/1cup
Frozen berries (any type)	250g/1 cup
Whey protein isolate (16-40 grams)	1 serving

The way to add variety is to switch the fruit from time to time; however, berries are the highest in antioxidants and lowest on the glycemic index. (More on the glycemic index is available in the chapter on Nutrition Basics.) Be sure to avoid bananas until the maintenance phase.

The protein powder you choose to use should contain no artificial sweeteners, artificial flavors, artificial colors, fillers, or preservatives. The only acceptable sweetener is Stevia or Stevia leaf. Stevia is a natural product and has been shown to be risk free, but I don't recommend it for weight loss. Part of this program is to withdraw from the addiction of sweet tasting foods. If possible, use an unflavored protein and let the natural, moderately-sweet taste of the fruit or berries impart the flavor.

Whey Protein Isolate

Whey protein isolate should always be used as it is a high quality protein and is easily digested. It has no lactose, so even those who are lactose intolerant can consume it. Whey protein concentrate is cheaper, but it contains lactose and will give lactose intolerant people problems.

Casein Protein

A slow digesting casein protein or whey isolate and casein blend would be excellent as well, but, during the writing of this book, none were available without artificial sweeteners added.

Soy Protein

Soy protein does not have a complete complement of amino acids making it inferior as a protein source.

Digestive Enzymes

Some brands of protein powder contain an enzyme blend to help digestion. Enzymes added may include: protease, lactase, amylase, papain, and bromelain. Any of these additions are a good thing.

An unflavored product means more protein and less filler.

Whey protein is not really a supplement; just another food. Think of whey protein powder as a chicken breast without the zinc and B vitamins. Protein powder has the same basic nutrition as chicken, but with the convenience of not having to be cooked.

Fast Meal Ideas

Get Lean Eggs with Vegetables

Sauté broccoli, onion, red/yellow peppers, and mushrooms in a small amount of olive oil. When the vegetables are almost finished cooking, stir in 2-4 beaten eggs. Scramble until eggs are cooked. Serve immediately. Garnish with salsa if desired.

Get Lean Chili Con Carne

Brown some extra lean ground beef. Sauté mushrooms and onions in the same pan. (You won't need to add any additional oil.) Put the beef, onions, and mushrooms into your crock pot or slow cooker. Add two cans of diced tomatoes. Add diced yellow peppers, sliced mushrooms, and chili powder to taste. Set the slow cooker on low for 8-12 hours. Fat burning chili!

Get Lean Chicken Soup / Stew

This is a very fast meal for those short on time. Cut up a pre-cooked chicken breast. Place the chicken breast in a microwave safe container. Add a full can of vegetable-based soup, preferably organic. Microwave and serve.

Get Lean Spaghetti

This is a spaghetti and meat sauce made with spaghetti squash instead of pasta. Make the spaghetti sauce as you always would. You can use stewed tomatoes, tomato paste, mushrooms, green pepper, onion, spices, and browned ground beef. You can make meat balls if you wish. The replacement for the pasta will be spaghetti squash. You can really fool yourself into thinking you're eating pasta. To cook, simply cut the spaghetti squash in half and place both halves face down on a 9x13 pan or a cookie sheet. Bake for about one hour at 350F (possibly longer, depending on the size). Cook until tender. When cooked, turn over and use a fork to strip out the tender, pasta-like squash. Plate a fist sized portion of squash with a fist sized portion of meat sauce. Meat should be about 50% of the sauce, giving you an optimal portion of one palm of protein from the ground beef.

Get Lean Lamb Shank Stew

A lamb shank has about 4-5oz of meat on it, making it the right size for most people. Cook the lamb shanks in a slow cooker overnight (on low for 8-10 hours) with diced tomatoes, sliced mushrooms, diced green peppers, chopped celery, and thinly sliced onions. Use ample coriander and cumin to taste. I love meals that cook themselves. Just cut up the vegetables and add them to the crock-pot. Add the meat. Add spices. In several hours, you'll have delicious hearty stew.

Staying on this phase permanently

It should be noted that there is nothing wrong with staying on the rapid weight loss phase indefinitely. Some of my clients like eating this way and continue to do so. They sometimes eat higher quantities of food than suggested in the rapid weight loss phase, but some never go back to eating any starchy tubers and continue to avoid grains, refined carbohydrates, and processed foods. This is a very healthy diet when followed for life.

Abs

For most people, a flat stomach is all they really want; however, some won't be satisfied unless they can see their abdominal muscles. People who have an underwear model type midsection eat similarly to the Rapid Weight Loss Phase 100% of the time. Abs or six-pack type stomachs come from continuous eating, similar to the Rapid Weight Loss Phase. Permanent eating in this structured way is unrealistic for most people. For individuals not satisfied with a flat stomach and who want to see significant definition, you will need to follow the above program indefinitely. The trainers I work with that have very defined bodies either do it with a moderate amount of strength training, cardiovascular training, and a diet similar to the diet above or they do it with an eating system similar to the maintenance phase, but they must do a huge amount of exercise as well.

To have defined abs, you must have the following:

1. A very low amount of body-fat between the abdominal muscles and the skin, so the muscle can be seen.

2. A very low overall body-fat percentage.
5-12% for men
10-18% for women

3. Very strong, muscular abdominal muscles projecting out from between the transverse intersections. (The lines that separate the abs into blocks are called transverse intersections.) Weaker abdominal muscles will have a flatter appearance.

To get defined abs, you must follow these steps:

1. Stay on the RWL phase until you can see all the abdominal definition you want and then continue to eat this way for life, 95 to 99% of the time. The portion size of protein may need to be increased in your diet to help the body recover from the intense exercise sessions required.
2. Use weights when training your midsection. Crunches, sit-ups, and other ab exercises with added weight create hypertrophy (muscle growth) necessary for the abs to be seen through the skin.
3. Do cardiovascular activity. This depends entirely on you. Some can get away with doing much less cardiovascular activity than others and still maintain a toned midsection. You will find out the necessary amount of activity required for your body through trial and error.

Psychological Factors

There are two main psychological barriers to weight loss:

a) Focus and association on the pleasure of unhealthy food
b) Panic due to lack of food

Focus involves where your mind is directed. If you think about how good a food will taste, you'll probably have trouble stopping yourself from eating it. If you focus on how terrible a food is for you, it will be easier to avoid it. Focus on how refined foods will make you feel: sluggish, tired, and scatterbrained. Focus on how a large portion of pasta will literally force the body to store fat due to high levels of insulin. Sometimes, associations about how horrible you will feel after eating a certain food can be motivating. Others will concentrate on how unhealthy a food is. For these people, knowing how high sugar consumption reduces effectiveness of the immune system will keep people on a path to a leaner body. Other people stay away from unhealthy foods or large portion sizes due to vanity-based associations. They focus on how eating sugar, flour products, and colas will cause them to gain body fat. When you are in a donut shop, focus on the fact that donuts will cause you to gain weight (or, at the least, prevent you from losing weight).

Cola will make you fat. Cola tastes good. Both are true, but the one you chose to focus on will determine your behavior. Focus on the detrimental effects unhealthy food has and you will find it easy to stop eating those foods.

You can also think about the many benefits of healthy foods when you are eating them. This may motivate you to eat and enjoy the healthiest foods more often. When you eat a healthy GLH meal, feel free to congratulate yourself for feeding your body what it needs to be healthy and lean.

The other psychological factor affecting weight loss is a state of panic often associated with a lack of food. If the body thinks you are starving, willpower won't work for very long. This is about survival.

To counteract this panic feeling, eat something every three hours. Never miss a meal or a snack. Make sure you eat enough food so that you aren't ravenous by your next meal. If you feel like you're starving, then you will likely panic and either eat the wrong foods or simply eat too much food.

Chapter 4: FAQ

Sometimes, questions have been voiced during the program by clients repeatedly. These may be questions you have as well, so they've been included here for your review.

Q: *It's too hard. What should I do?*
A: Stick with it! A change affecting your lifestyle is always hard. Albert Einstein said, "Insanity is doing the same thing over and over again but expecting a different result." You must change your lifestyle radically and permanently to lose weight as well as keep it off. Your lifestyle, thus far, has given you the body you currently have and unless you are willing to change, your body won't. Eating the same things that you eat now will only maintain the body you have now. No food tastes as good as how good having a healthy, fit, and lean body makes you feel. Stick with the program and your taste for wholesome foods will develop, slowly but surely, if you stick with it. Soon, usually after about a month of following the GLH program, the old sweet foods you craved will actually taste bad!

Q: *I'm hungry! What should I do?*
A: Snack on raw almonds. Other nuts are acceptable, too, but avoid peanuts as they are not real nuts. Peanuts are actually legumes and are therefore higher in phytates/phytic acid, which can deplete minerals. (Almonds, walnuts, and Brazil nuts are the healthiest.) Add one small handful of almonds to the two snacks between meals, so you'll be eating fruit and nuts at each snack. If you stop losing weight, cut back to only having almonds with the morning snack. Evaluate your hunger. Do you have cravings or are you really hungry? Perhaps, you are thirsty? Does drinking water help curb these cravings?

Q: I'm hungry and I can't eat nuts.

(Or) I'm hungry and I don't like nuts. What should I do?

A: Eat a bit more protein at each meal. Eat more than a palm. This may help. Again, evaluate your progress. Are you craving foods that are not on the system or are you really hungry?

Q: I've just started the program and I have a slight headache. Is this normal?

A: Addiction to refined carbohydrates can sometimes have withdrawal symptoms similar to stopping caffeine intake. This is normal. In one to two days, the headache will usually fade away. **(If you have what seems like a severe headache or your headache lasts longer than what you consider normal, please use common sense. See your physician immediately!)**

Q: I have low energy. Why?

A: This is not uncommon. Some people have this lethargic feeling for one to three days as the body gets used to the program. (You will not be in ketosis as the carbohydrate intake is not as low as low carbohydrate diets. Ketosis happens when carbohydrate intake is very low.)

Q: I'm losing weight but I can't seem to lose the fat around my midsection/thighs/backside (or any other problem area). What should I do?

A: Stick with it! We all put on fat in different places and most of this fat placement is genetic. The more time you spend on the program, the less troubling your trouble spots will look!

Q: I can't seem to lose the fat around my midsection only. What should I do?

A: Stress is likely holding you back! Are you stressed? The stress hormone, cortisol, will make your body hold more abdominal fat. Take a close look at your lifestyle. Tackle the problem at the source. Change your stress levels by learning how to deal with stress better and you will lose midsection fat. Consider yoga, mediation, or just take a little time for yourself every day. Exercise of any sort is a great way to relieve stress.

Q: *I'm Pregnant. What should I do?*

A: Consult your doctor. **This is not a time to focus on weight loss. Instead, focus on eating a healthy diet and reducing weight after the baby is born and breastfeeding has been completed.** Begin taking a high quality prenatal vitamin/mineral/antioxidant formula with folic acid as soon as possible Better yet, get on the prenatal supplements six months before getting pregnant.

Q: *I'm breastfeeding. What should I do differently?*

A: Refer to the above Q&A entry. You should still be on the prenatal vitamins.

Q: *I exercise more than the ½ hour that you recommend. Do I need more food than the Rapid Weight Loss phase?*

A: Maybe. Directly after a long hard workout, eat an extra fist sized portion of fruit to replenish your glycogen stores. (Glycogen is the stored sugar in muscles.)

Q: *I do a lot of weight training. Do I need more protein and/or carbo-hydrates?*

A: Maybe. If you do weight training to gain muscle mass, follow the template below. The protein intake is higher, to offset the breakdown of muscle protein from a high amount of weight training. This diet requires more planning and cooking, but bodybuilders and strength athletes should consider using this system.

Meal 1   Protein – palm sized portion or Nutrition Shake
             Fruit – palm sized portion
             Yogurt – palm sized portion

  Snack   Protein – palm sized portion
             Vegetables – unlimited

Meal 2   Protein – palm sized portion
             Vegetables – unlimited

  Snack – post workout
             Protein – palm sized portion
             Fruit – fist sized portion x2

Meal 3   Protein – palm sized portion
          Vegetables – unlimited

Q: *I'm a vegetarian. How can I make the system work for me?*
A: This program simply will not work as well for strict vegetarians. Humans evolved to eat meat and fish. That is why we have smaller abdomens than chimpanzees (our closest primate relative). The chimpanzee diet is higher in plant material than the human diet and their gastrointestinal tract is longer, to better digest more plant matter. However, chimps also eat meat. Meat accounts for about 5-30% of their diet, depending on what area they live in. Try these protein sources if you chose not to eat meat for cultural, religious, or ethical reasons:

1. Cottage cheese
2. Hard Cheeses
3. Almonds, nuts, and nut butter
4. Plain yogurt
5. Tofu, tempe, and other soy products and legumes
   such as lentils, beans, and chickpeas.
   (None of these sources are predominantly protein. They
   are either a mix of fat and protein or a mix of carbohydrate
   and protein. Example: Yogurt is 40:60 ratio of protein to
   carbohydrates.)

If you don't eat meat for health reasons, because you are worried about the injected hormones, antibiotics, and pesticide residue from feed, switch to organic meats. Certified organic meats do not contain hormones, antibiotics, and cannot have mad cow disease. Mad cow disease is derived from feeding cows animal byproducts (sheep, cows, chickens, and etc.). Certified organic beef is never fed animal byproducts.

If you're a vegetarian because of ethical reasons, consider how certi-fied organic livestock is treated much more humanely than conven-tional farming methods. Certified organic chicken must be free range, as well as organic eggs harvested from free range chickens, and so forth.

Q: *What if I'm in a situation where I must eat fast food?*
A: Never eat fast food. But, if you're ever in a situation where there

is truly no choice and you have to eat fast food, never get the combo. There is no place in any healthy diet for soft drinks and French fries. (Remember this rule, even during the maintenance phase!) Depending on the size of the fries and drink, they could easily triple the calories of the meal! Although this strategy is not ideal, if there is no other choice, eat the sandwich, burger, grilled chicken sandwich, taco, or whatever is available with a bottle of water and start planning for your next nutritious GLH meal.

Q: *I broke even this week. I didn't lose weight or gain any weight. Why?*
A: This usually only happens when you don't follow the program 100%. But, this is a good lesson. Now you have an idea of how well you have to eat just to maintain your bodyweight. If you cheated twice, then you may be able to get away with it during the maintenance phase. If you had two whole bad days of eating and didn't gain weight, consider yourself lucky.

Q: *I broke even this week and I didn't cheat. I followed the program exactly as written. Why?*
A: This sometimes happens, but it won't happen two weeks in a row. The body will catch-up next week and, quite likely, you'll lose extra weight. Weight loss is rarely linear; the body tends to shed a couple of pounds in a couple of days and then stabilize for a few days. Stay vigilant.

Q: *What if I miss a meal or snack?*
A: Don't. The program is designed with very specific quantities. By missing or skipping snacks and meals, you'll be really hungry and you might possibly make bad food choices. Please avoid falling into this bad habit. Your body may also be tricked into thinking it's starving, slowing your metabolism in preparation for the lack of food.

Q: *I'm dying for sweets after dinner.*
A: After dinner, try eating berries or fruit as desert. Keep the portion small. Palm sized at the maximum. Avoid this if possible. Remember, you need to get used to this new way of eating if you're really serious about getting lean and staying lean.

Q: *My bowel movements are less regular on this program. What can I do?*

A: This shouldn't be the case as you are starting to eat more fiber than ever before from a plethora of high fiber fruits and vegetables. Sometimes, however, any change in diet has a negative effect on elimination. There are a few things you can try to help relieve/regulate the situation.

1. Eat more high fiber vegetables.
2. Drink more water.
3. Eat more apples and pears for snacks.
4. Supplement your diet with Psyillium husks. This will work wonders for you. Psyillium is a natural grain-based fiber source that is very high in soluble fiber. Take 1 tbsp daily in a glass of water followed by a second glass of water. If you do not drink enough water when you take psyillium, you will get the opposite effect. It can act as a plug and create constipation. If you use psyillium, you MUST drink lots of water.

Q: *Why are there no specific exercises recommended with the GLH system?*

A: With exercise, form (biomechanics) is everything. You cannot learn how to perform the proper execution of various exercises from reading a book. Turn to a competent certified personal trainer to show you how to exercise correctly and safely. Someone needs to watch you perform an exercise to see if you are getting it right. There are fitness centers around the globe filled with people wasting their time performing exercises incorrectly. Best case scenario, these people wasted their time. Worst case scenario, they get hurt or create muscle imbalances which could lead to a future injury. If you plan to add various forms of exercise to your change in lifestyle, and I recommend that you do, work with a professional who can ensure you are safely and effectively working out.

Q: *I'm stuck and I only have five more pounds to lose. What should I do?*

A: With the last five pounds, sometimes it is necessary to cut fruit completely out of your diet for two weeks. Do this only for two to three weeks at a time. Eat a handful of almonds at the mid afternoon and midmorning snack. Eat protein and vegetables for breakfast, lunch, and dinner. Yes, breakfast will contain lots of protein and vegetables as well. Following this should shed the last five to ten pounds off easily.

If the above doesn't work, however, evaluate exactly what you're eating and doing. Are you having too much salad dressing? Are you exercising for at least 30 minutes a day?

Some people have to exercise more to get the last 5-10 pounds off. At this point, you may need to increase your activity to one hour a day.

Q: The food on this program is expensive! Is it really worth the added expense?
A: The added expense is totally worth it. Healthy foods give the body unparalleled vitality. Fresh produce and quality protein is more expensive than unhealthy processed foods, but it is also far higher in vitamins, minerals, and fiber. Many people who eat processed food take a multi-vitamin and/or a multi-mineral supplement to balance what is missing from their nutrient poor diet. This will not work nearly as well as eating a healthy diet. The multi-vitamin will not have the enzymes of raw produce and it will not have the level of fiber your body needs. Processed foods are almost always higher on the glycemic index, so they lead to weight gain. When you add up the cost of trying to add supplements to a poor diet, a healthy diet of whole, unprocessed foods is cheaper than fast food and supplements. The better you eat the fewer supplements you'll need.

Consider the cost of heath care. If you eat more fast food, you're going to be more at risk for various diseases. Health care is expensive, but the best quality organic produce is relatively cheap.

Q: I cheated this week, but only on 1 bran muffin and a handful of candy. Why did I not lose any weight?
A: For most people the rapid weight loss phase must be followed 100% to get weight loss; if not, it's just a pretty healthy diet.

Q: This does not seem like a normal diet. Is it really healthy?
A: Yes, this is a very healthy diet. And no, it is not normal! The Standard American Diet (SAD) has made over 50% of the North American

population overweight. People who follow SAD as their diet are often overweight or have other health problems.

Q: *Why is there no starch in the program?*
A: Starch effectively stops weight loss. There's no starch in this program to allow you to break your addiction to starchy foods. Many people who are not eaters of sweets still get an amazing amount of sugar in their diet. A baked potato has the equivalent of 20-30 teaspoons of sugar. However, even though the GLH system is low in starch, the diet is fairly high in carbohydrates from the equivalent of 6 to 9 servings of fruit and 6 to 16 servings of vegetables per day. There is also a great deal of carbohydrate in the suggested servings of yogurt.

Q: *Should I write down what I'm eating in a food log or food journal?*
A: For many people, this is a helpful activity. If you're serious about losing weight, you will want to do this. A food log is even included in this book to help you get started. When progress starts to slow for anyone, they should begin writing everything they eat down. There is something about writing down exactly what is eaten that helps people strictly adhere to the program.

Q: *What about "cheat days" or "cheat meals" - where you can diverge from the program for a period of time?*
A: On this program, cheating is only allowed on the maintenance phase. You probably won't lose weight very fast on the Rapid Weight Loss phase if you cheat. By cheating, you only cheat yourself.

Q: *Why are there no grains on the Rapid Weight Loss Phase?*
A: The human body evolved over millions of years to thrive best on a hunt and gather model of diet. Grains were not a part of the human diet for the first 2 million years. Imagine for a moment that you are a Paleolithic person. Are you going to gather food as small as individual grains in order to survive? Research shows that Paleolithic people hunted animals, fished, and gathered nuts, fruits, and vegetables for food. Grains were not harvested until agriculture first started, around 10,000 years ago. Grains are a relatively new food, so our bodies have not learned how to deal well with them yet.

There is evidence showing that grains and legumes may not be an ideal food source for humans. Grains and legumes contain phytates, which bond to minerals and remove their nutritional value. Phytates can drain minerals from the human body.

Limiting all grain consumption and removing all bakery items from your diet is an important step to good health and permanent weight management.

Q: *How do I punch up the flavor?*

A: Here's how:

Some ways to boost flavor and add taste:

• Grill veggies on the BBQ (brushed with a small amount of olive oil)

• BBQ your protein sources (but never char the food as this creates carcinogenic properties)

• Use a variety of dry herbs and spices

• Cook with fresh herbs

• Use salsa (use brands without sugar, such as Pace and some organic varieties)

• Add garlic

• Use fresh lemon

• Grill mushrooms

• Sautéed onion

• Any sauce that is vegetable based and has no sugar is acceptable.

• Any dressing or sauce made with cold pressed oil / expeller pressed oil/extra virgin oil is good in moderation. (limit to 1tsp per 100 pounds of bodyweight per meal)

Q: *Fruit and vegetables can be eaten raw, so preparation is sometimes as simple as washing and eating. Protein foods (other than protein powder) need to be cooked and can take considerable amounts of time. I don't have time, what can I do?*

A: Cook in bulk. Cook ahead. Every Sunday night, bake lots of protein to eat over the next week. Bake a tray of chicken breasts, a tray of lean turkey sausages, a tray of fresh fish, beef, or whatever else you feel like. Cook at least 2-3 sources of protein so you don't get bored. Make enough for every meal of the week. Put half in the fridge and half in the freezer to be defrosted mid-week. Now you have protein on demand, and all you have to do is just heat and serve. (Keep cooked food in the refrigerator for no longer than 3 days.)

The Maintenance Phase - How to keep it off Forever

Congratulations! You have worked hard and lost all of the weight you wanted to lose and, now, you want to learn how to keep it off.

This is the most important phase. You need to follow a lifestyle with dietary habits the body can stay lean on. Lots of people are a bit nervous at this time, because some have successfully lost weight before and gained it all back. The maintenance program is not very different from the rapid weight loss phase. The major change to the Get Lean and Healthy system at this phase is the inclusion of low fiber/high starch carbohydrate foods. These foods are not as healthy as their high fiber cousins, because they are generally lower in vitamins, minerals, and fiber. But, we don't want to deny you these foods forever. Low fiber/high starch carbohydrates, such as brown rice and potatoes, can trigger the body to store fat and must always be eaten as a palm sized portion and with a palm sized protein food.

Maintanance Meal

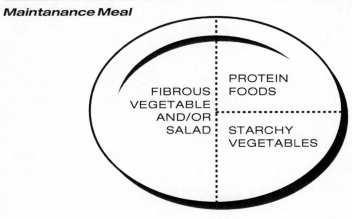

FIBROUS VEGETABLE AND/OR SALAD

PROTEIN FOODS

STARCHY VEGETABLES

Starchy Carbohydrate Sources: (Maintenance Phase Only)

Brown rice, whole grains, carrots, parsnips, potatoes, oatmeal, any type of squash, yams, chickpeas, kidney beans, or any other type of legumes can now be consumed.

Always stick to whole grains when eating rice, oats, wheat, and other grains. Whole grains contain all the vitamins, minerals, and fiber that nature intended. Any refined grains (white rice, white bread, etc.) contain primarily starch. Also, most of the vitamins and fiber have been removed during the processing of the food.

Bread can now be eaten; however, limit intake to a palm sized portion. (Usually this would be 1 slice, possibly 2 if you're a very tall person or if it is rye bread.) Also, limit how often you eat bread as those who eat it too often tend to put on weight. Whole grain bread is preferred and, if you're really interested in keeping the weight off, stick with whole grain rye bread. Rye is lower on the glycemic index than most other whole grains, so it holds less potential to stimulate the body to store fat. Real rye bread has whole grain rye flour as the first ingredient. If the first ingredient is enriched flour or wheat flour, consider the product white bread and avoid it.

Remember to keep the starch portions palm sized or less, or you'll start gaining the weight back.

Commit now to healthy eating and exercise, because it will take a lifelong commitment to stay lean.

Maintenance Program Outline (1300 – 3000Kcal)

Meal 1   Protein – palm sized portion or Nutrition Shake
               Fruit – palm sized portion   - 1 cup plain yogurt
               Yogurt – palm sized portion   - 1 cup frozen berries
                                           - ½ cup water
                                         - ½ - *1 banana*
                                         - 1 scoop whey protein
                                            isolate
                                         Blend and enjoy.

Snack   Fruit – fist sized portion *or* a handful of raw almonds

Meal 2   Protein – palm sized portion
***Starchy vegetables, whole grains, or legumes –
palm sized portion***
Fibrous vegetables – unlimited

Snack   Fruit – fist sized portion *or* a handful of raw almonds

Meal 3   Protein – palm sized portion
***Starchy vegetables, whole grains, or legumes –
palm sized portion***
Fibrous vegetables – unlimited

Sample Menus:

Menu A

Meal 1   Poached eggs
Whole grain rye toast with butter
Fresh berries

Snack   1 Large orange

Meal 2   Chicken leg
Salad
Brown rice

Snack   Handful of raw almonds

Meal 3   Lamb chops
Sweet potato
Large greek salad

Menu B

Meal 1   Super Oatmeal (Plain, unsweetened oatmeal with cinnamon and raisins; mix unflavored whey protein powder into the cooked oatmeal. Let the cooked oats cool a bit before putting in the protein or the protein will clump.)

Snack   1 handful of Brazil nuts

Meal 2   Bison burger
Rye bread
2-3 cups of raw vegetables

Snack   1 Pear

Meal 3   Grilled fish
Brown rice
Grilled vegetables
Mixed baby greens with olive oil, red wine vinegar,
and Dijon mustard

Maintenance Foods

Below are some very healthy foods that can only be eaten during the maintenance phase. Stay clear of these foods if you are trying to lose weight.

Healthy Starchy Carbohydrate Foods
(Maintenance phase only! Eat in moderation due to high amounts of carbohydrates and little fiber.)

Grains - Maintenance Phase Only
* Barley
* Buckwheat
* Millet
* Oats
* Rice, brown
* Rye
* Spelt
* Wheat

Beans and Legumes – Maintenance Phase Only
* Black beans
* Garbanzo beans
* Kidney beans
* Lentils

- Lima beans
- Miso
- Navy beans
- Soybeans
- Tempeh
- Tofu

(Limit your consumption of unsprouted grains and legumes to three servings a week because of phytates. There is more information on the detrimental effects of phytates in the 30 Days to Optimal Nutrition chapter. Eat as many sprouted grains and legumes as you wish.)

Starchy Vegetables – Maintenance Phase Only
- Beets
- Carrots
- Potatoes
- Sweet Potatoes
- Yams

Low Fiber Fruit – Maintenance Phase Only
- Banana
- Dried fruit (any)

Stay Lean Nutrition Shakes

Your nutrition shakes can now have one half to one full banana, depending on the size of your body and the size of the banana. The taste and texture will be much better, but monitor your weight carefully. Bananas can make you gain weight. If you start to put on weight, omit the banana. You can now also add nut butter, such as almond butter, to your shakes. One tablespoon can be added per shake to add fiber and essential fatty acids (EFAs). The nut butter goes well with bananas, but does not compliment the berries.

Blend and enjoy the following ingredients:

Stay Lean Recipe 1: Berry Banana

1. Water	250ml/1 cup
2. Yogurt (plain /unsweetened)	250g/1cup
3. Frozen berries (any type)	250g/1 cup
4. Whey protein isolate (16-40 grams)	1 serving
5. Banana	½ to 1 fruit

Stay Lean Recipe 2: **Almond Banana**

1. Water	250ml/1 cup
2. Yogurt (plain /unsweetened)	250g/1cup
3. Almond butter	1tbsp
4. Whey protein isolate (16-40 grams)	1 serving
5. Banana	½ to 1 fruit

The 90% Rule

Follow *The 90% Rule*. You are going to stray from this mechanical system of eating once in a while – it is inevitable. Eat using this main-tenance system 90% of the time and let yourself indulge the remaining 10% of the time. You can really eat anything 10% of the time; however, try to keep these indulgences down to 10% at maximum. **If you go back to the way you ate before, you'll gain all the weight back, guaranteed!**

Healthy Nutrition 101

As a Registered Holistic Nutritionist, my focus is on health first. An effective weight loss diet that doesn't improve overall health is not acceptable to me, nor should it be acceptable to you. The following will help you acquire some basic strategies for getting the most from your nutrition.

I have been studying nutrition for most of my life. I started my informal study at 14 years of age. Soon after, I gave up drinking pop and eating French fries. Can you imagine a teenager who refuses to eat fried foods and won't drink a sip of cola? That was me. I've studied nutrition constantly for almost 20 years, so my depth of knowledge is great; however, this will only be a very brief and very concise look at the basics.

Nutrition is the study of nutrients, the building blocks of food. These building blocks are divided into two broad categories: macronutrients and micronutrients. Macronutrients are big nutrients and micronutrients are small nutrients.

Macronutrients

There are only 4 types of macronutrients: water, carbohydrates, proteins, and fat. All food is made up of one or more types of these big components.

1. *Protein*
2. *Fat / Oils*
3. *Carbohydrates*
4. *Water*

Examples:

> Fruit = water + carbohydrates
> Meat = protein + fat
> Yogurt = protein + fat + water + carbohydrates

Macronutrients provide energy for the body. They also create structure for tissues in the body. The body is actually made out of macronutrients, so the old saying really is true -- you literally are what you eat.

Micronutrients

There are only two types of micronutrients: vitamins and minerals. (In reality, it is slightly more complex than this, but for our purposes, consider this to be true.)   *1. Vitamins*
                                             2. Minerals

Vitamins act as catalysts and provide assistance for metabolic transitions in the body. They are like tools by helping build as well as breakdown things in our body. Vitamins also release energy.

Minerals create tissue structure by adding rigidity to bones and teeth. Like vitamins, minerals also help with many body processes.

Antioxidants, vitamins and minerals such as A, C, E, zinc, selenium, prevent the body from breaking down from free radical damage. They cannot stop aging, but they can slow down the overall effects, somewhat.

All "whole food" contains micronutrients. (Whole food, in this context, means unprocessed food.) Processed food may or may not contain micronutrients, depending on how it has been processed.

Do you ever wonder why white flour is called "enriched wheat flour"? (Which serves to make it sound healthier than it really is.) When flour is processed, the manufacturer takes out the husk and the germ, leaving only the starch, which is bleached to remove the color. This process takes out all the vitamins. In the past, people who obtained most of their nutrients from bread risked vitamin deficiency diseases.

The manufacturers of white flour were then forced by governments to add some vitamins back into their white bread and pasta mixes to stop the occurrence of vitamin deficiency diseases. I've eaten white bread a few times since I was 14, but I avoid it whenever I can, In fact, I rarely consume bread at all, but if I do, it's from a whole grain source. (When I want to see deep cuts in my abs, I always cut out bread altogether - at least for a few weeks.)

Eat a wide variety of fruits and vegetables to get your daily requirements of vitamins and minerals.

Now we will go into a little more depth.

More on Macronutrients

Each type of macronutrient (protein, fat, carbohydrate, and water) can be broken down further into different categories.

Fats / Oils
There are four basic types of fats: saturated, monounsaturated, polyunsaturated, and trans-fats. The first three types are healthy, as long as you are getting balance of all three.

Polyunsaturated Fats
- Very healthy.
- Unstable, cannot be used for cooking. High temperatures will break down oil into harmful trans-fats.
- Improves cholesterol ratio.
- Sources: Fish, nuts, flax seeds.
- Liquid at room temperature.

Monounsaturated Fats
- Very Healthy.
- Somewhat stable, can be cooked with at moderate temperature. Very high temperatures will break down oil into harmful trans-fats.
- Improves cholesterol ratio.
- Sources: Olive oil, canola oil, avocado, nuts.
- Liquid at room temperature.

Saturated Fats

- Healthy in moderation.
- Very stable, can be cooked with at high temperature.
- Increases harmful LDL cholesterol, but no reduction of HDL.
- Sources: Butter, beef, chicken, dairy, coconut oil.
- Solid at room temperature.

Trans-fats (hydrogenated fats)

- Very unhealthy.
- Stable.
- Very detrimental to cholesterol and overall health. Ten times more dangerous than saturated fats.
- Sources: Margarine, baked goods, crackers, french-fries, some children's foods, chips. (Most, but not all of the above, contain trans-fats; it depends on the manufacturer.)
- Solid at room temperature.

Some would say that saturated fats are as bad as trans-fats. This is not true -- if eaten in moderation. Saturated fats come primarily from milk, cheese, beef, and eggs. A reasonable amount of saturated fat would include a palm sized portion of beef for two meals a week, dairy a few times a week (5-10), and up to six eggs a week (more if omega 3 eggs).

Monounsaturated and polyunsaturated fats are found in foods such as fish, almonds, and olive oil. Eat more of these fats. Foods containing these oils will help defend against heart disease by increasing your good cholesterol (HDL) and lowering your bad cholesterol (LDL). (Over simplifications like "good" and "bad" are misleading. It's really all about balance. You would die with a complete absence of bad cholesterol, so it's not really bad unless it gets too high.) Entire books have been written lately about the positive benefits of quality fats.

Protein

All protein is made up of 22 amino acids. These 22 amino acids are building blocks to make different types of protein. Some of these 22 amino acids can be manufactured by the body; eight cannot.

Meat and dairy contain all eight amino acids the body cannot make. These eight amino acids are called the essential amino acids. Plant-based sources of protein do not contain all eight of these essential amino acids. Plant-based foods must be combined to make up for the missing amino acids. For example, a grain must be eaten with a legume to get all eight essential amino acids. Even when combined, plant-based foods are lower in overall protein, so they are still a relatively poor choice when choosing a protein food.

The protein foods below are ranked based upon quality, using the protein efficiency ratio (PER). The PER ranks protein sources based upon how well they provide a complement of amino acids deemed ideal for human consumption.

Further below, protein sources are ranked against the quantity of protein per 100 grams.

Protein Efficiency Ratio (PER)

Higher Quality Protein Sources – Meat, Fish, Dairy
- Egg — 3.8
- Fish — 3.6
- Beef — 3.2
- Whey Protein Isolate — 3.2
- Milk — 2.8
- Cheese — 2.8

Lower Quality Protein Sources – Plant-based
- Soy — 2.3
- Oats — 2.2
- Lentils — 1.7
- Chickpeas — 1.7
- Peanuts — 1.7
- Whole Wheat — 1.5
- Navy Beans — 1.2
- White Bread — 1.0
- Almonds — 0.4

The plant-based protein sources are missing 1 or more of the eight essential amino acids. Therefore they are considered incomplete protein sources.

Quantity of Protein in Grams /100 grams of food (unless stated)

Values are approximate due to the varying fat content of meats and cheeses. Depending on the source, variations in protein content can also be seen in grains, nuts, and beans.

- Whey Protein Isolate (40 grams)   37
- Beef   28
- Chicken   25
- Fish   24
- Eggs (2)   13
- Soybeans   12
- Tofu – Regular/Extra Firm   8/16
- Lentils   8
- Navy Beans   8
- Chickpeas   8
- Milk (1 glass)   7
- Cheese (1oz)   7
- Peanuts (1oz)   7
- Almonds (1oz, 23 Almonds)   6
- Cooked Brown Rice   3
- Cooked Oats   2
- Whole Wheat (1 slice)   2
- White Bread (1 slice)   2

Carbohydrates

There are two types of carbohydrates: simple and complex. Simple carbohydrates are also called sugars. Complex carbohydrates are sometimes called starches.

1. Simple Carbohydrates (Sugars)
2. Complex Carbohydrates (Starches)

It was once thought that complex carbohydrates were better, because it was thought that they digested slower. Not true. The digestion of carbohydrates starts in your mouth, so by the time most complex carbohydrate foods hit your stomach, they are already broken down into sugar.

As stated before, carbohydrate-rich foods that contain a lot of fiber are assimilated more slowly, leading to sustained energy and less fat storage. It doesn't matter whether the carbohydrates are simple or complex; what matters is how much fiber the food contains.

Glycemic Index (GI)

To help us better understand nutrition, foods are ranked on the glycemic index (GI) which calculates how fast blood sugar rises after a food is eaten. This is the real way to judge how good a carbohydrate is at giving sustained energy. Foods higher on the GI spike blood sugar levels, leading to fat storage and less energy. Foods lower on the glycemic index are better, leading to sustained energy and more fat burning.

So, why isn't there a 10 page GI listed in this book for you to use in referencing all the carbohydrate foods that you eat? There is a much simpler way to determine the best carbohydrates to eat. All you need to know is the amount of fiber in the food as relative to the total digestible carbohydrate to know where the food falls on the GI.

The higher the fiber of a food, the lower the food will be on the GI. The greater the digestible carbohydrate (sugar and starch), the higher the food is on the GI. That is why during the Rapid Weight Loss phase you only eat high fiber, lower carbohydrate vegetables and fruit. By eating only high fiber carbohydrates, you automatically eat only low GI foods.

A rating of 0 on the index means that your blood sugar did not increase at all. A rating of 100 on the GI means that the food increased your blood sugar at the same rate as eating 100 grams of sugar. The lower the GI, the more fat burning; the higher the GI, the more fat storage.

Example of one fruit and one vegetable:

Food	GI Rating (0-100)
Not eaten on RWL phase of GLH	
• Baked Potato	85
• Banana	62

Food	**GI Rating (0-100)**
Eaten on RWL phase of GLH	
• Broccoli	15
• Apple	34

More on Micronutrients

Micronutrients are abundant in whole, unrefined foods. Processed foods contain little micronutrients. Eating unprocessed foods from a variety of sources will ensure you get adequate vitamins and minerals. Remember that certain foods are higher than others in micronutrients. The recommended foods in this book have the highest micronutrients of any widely available foods.

Chapter 7: 30 Days to Optimal Nutrition

These are 30 changes you can make to get the most out of your nutrition and your body! Implement one a day or start on all 30 today, it doesn't matter as long as you do it. They all relate to good nutrition. Some should be followed on the maintenance phase, while others are appropriate to the Rapid Weight Loss phase. Some of these changes do not relate directly to weight loss, but help increase over-all health and vitality.

The information with an asterisk(*) beside it will directly help with weight loss. The rest will help with long-term weight loss goals by contributing to overall health, thereby allowing optimal efficiencies in your body.

1. Limit or Eliminate Refined Sugar*
2. Eat more Vegetables*
3. Replace Coffee with Green Tea*
4. Eliminate all Processed Meat
5. Improve your Digestion
6. Drink More Water*
7. Supplement with Fish Oil*
8. Take a Vitamin/Mineral Supplement*
9. Eat Organic
10. Eat Wild Fish, Avoid Farmed Fish
11. Eat less Soy Products
12. Eat only Sprouted Grains and Legumes
13. Consume Protein at every Meal*
14. Consume less Alcohol*
15. Avoid Artificial Sweeteners

16. Eliminate Preservatives
17. Eat more Raw Food
18. Eat more Whole Foods*
19. Eat more Fiber*
20. Avoid Trans-fats
21. Avoid Low Fat and Carbohydrate Foods
22. Eat more Antioxidant Rich Foods
23. Make Healthy Choices when Eating Out*
24. Exercise More*
25. Avoid Liquid Sugar – Juice and Cola*
26. Eat More Super-foods
27. Eat More Yogurt
28. Eat More Omega 3 Eggs*
29. Practice a Daily 12 Hour Liver Fast*
30. Be Aware of what You're Eating*

1. Limit or Eliminate Refined Sugar

Refined sugar can create obesity, heart disease, and type II diabetes. It has the potential to be as dangerous as smoking, if eaten in large enough quantities. Obesity-related diseases have eclipsed smoking as the leading cause of preventable death in North America. Why is refined sugar accepted, where as smoking is not? Limit exposure to sugar for health and, as a bonus, lose weight. Giving up sugar for life is one of the very best things you can do to stay lean for life.

Avoid:
- Cola
- BBQ Sauce
- Ketchup
- Candy
- Dessert
- Chocolate Bars
- Jams and Jellies

2. Eat more Vegetables

Vegetables (fibrous) are very high in antioxidants, micronutrients, and fiber. They will help you lose weight by just being low on the GI.

Vegetables are the number one food you can eat because of their high level of vitamins, minerals, antioxidants, and fiber. For optimal nutrition, vegetables should comprise half of what you eat.

3. Replace Coffee with Green Tea

Green tea has been clinically proven to help with weight loss. It is also beneficial because it contains high amounts of antioxidants. Green tea also has only 30% of the caffeine found in coffee.

Coffee can send your blood sugar on a roller coaster ride. Stable, consistent, blood sugar is necessary for sustained energy as well as for fat loss. Coffee is also very acidic. This acidity can lead to a draining of the minerals from the body, as minerals are used to buffer coffee's acidic effects.

Swap coffee for green tea and you'll lose weight quicker, have more consistent energy, and have better health.

If you don't like the taste of green tea, you can supplement your diet with green tea extract. This is one of very few weight loss supplements that work. Remember, what you eat is at least 10 times as important as the supplement you take. Think of it like this:

70% Nutrition
25% Exercise
5% Supplements

4. Eliminated All Processed (preserved) Meats

Most bacon, back bacon, lunch meats, and deli meats contain cancer causing preservatives.

CANCER!

Cook turkey breasts or small, lean roasts of beef, and cut off slices. They won't last as long in the fridge, but they won't contain added carcinogens.

5. Improve your Digestion

Feeling gassy or bloated? These suggestions may help.

1. Chew food thoroughly. There are no teeth in your stomach to break down large food particles. Also, the salivary enzyme amylase actually begins the digestion of carbohydrates in your mouth. Only food broken down fully can be assimilated by the body.

2. Eat slowly to prepare the body for food entering the digestive tract. Your body gets signals from your senses to start the digestion process. If you eat food quickly, without using your senses to taste it and smell it, your digestion will not be optimal. Digestion begins with the senses sensing food and the body responding by preparing to digest it. Also, and this is very important for weight management, eating slowly will allow the "full" signal to occur before you overeat.

3. Eat smaller meals more frequently to avoid overloading the digestive system.

4. Eat more soluble fiber. Soluble fiber, the kind found in apples, pears, other fruits, grains, and vegetables can cleanse the digestive system. While fiber does not have a direct effect on the digestion of food, it is good for the gastrointestinal tract. Soluble fiber coupled with an adequate intake of water can be very cleansing to the digestive system.

Excellent Sources:
- Psyllium Husks
- Flax Seeds
- Apples, pears, oranges, other fruits
- Nuts
- Oats, Oat bran
- Barley

5. Eat more raw foods. Foods heated above 118F have denatured or inactive enzymes. Raw foods have active enzymes and assist in digesting the meal eaten. Therefore, raw foods take demand off of the pancreas. The pancreas does not have to supply all the enzymes necessary for digestion.

6. Relax while eating. Being in a stressed condition or having your nervous system in a sympathetic state (fight or flight) will shut down the digestion process. All energy production goes to the most important systems. Stress to primitive humans usually meant a life or death situation, so we evolved to almost completely shut down digestion in times of stress. If you're eating at your desk, stressed to the point of smoke coming out of your ears, you're not digesting.

7. Reduce consumption of water or liquid with meals. Drink plenty of water between meals, but avoid excessive water with meals as it can reduce stomach acidity and lead to impaired protein digestion. (A good rule to follow is to drink water up until 30 minutes before a meal and start drinking again 30 minutes after a meal.)

8. Consider taking a digestive enzyme supplement. If, after doing the above suggestions for a couple of days your digestion is still not working well, consider taking enzymes. By supplementing temporarily with digestive enzymes, you will remove pressure from your pancreas to supply all the enzymes necessary to digest your food. Meals containing raw foods, such as salads, fruits, and raw vegetables, will usually require less supplemental enzymes, although not always. Below are three enzyme supplements suggestions that may be of additional help.

> 1. **Bromelain** – pineapple enzymes
> 2. **Papain** – papaya enzymes (As a general rule, eating more pineapple and papaya will help.)
> 3. **Pancreatic enzymes**
>   1. lipase – breakdown fat
>   2. protease – breakdown protein
>   3. amylase – breakdown carbohydrate

6. Drink More Water

As stated in the Rapid Weight Loss chapter, you should drink 1L (over four cups) for every 50 pounds of bodyweight per day. That is 4L (16 cups) for a 200 pound person. Start slowly and work up to this level of consumption. If you are inactive (and you shouldn't be), you won't need quite so much. You will need more when you are exposed to the heat and much more during exercise in hot weather.

7. Supplement with Fish Oil

Omega 3 (EPA and DHA)

Fat that helps you fight fat.

Omega 3 Essential Fatty Acids (EFAs) from a source such as fish oil or flax oil should be taken daily. Fish oil is best because it has more EPA and DHA. Fish oil also has shown to be more helpful with weight loss. Or, you can take an Omega 3, 6, 9 blend of polyunsaturated fatty acids; although omega 3 is the most important. EFAs are the most important supplements you can take. They help with skin problems, neurological disorders, the brain, and nerves. They can even help prevent heart disease. Omega 3 fatty acids can also help you lose weight. Fish oil is the best because the liver has to do the least amount of processing. The EPA & DHA are ready for use.

Fish oil should be pharmaceutical grade. Most fish is somewhat contaminated with mercury, which is toxic to brain tissue. Pharmaceutical grade fish oil is the most rigorously tested for contaminants. It doesn't matter which species of fish oil you use, but it must be pure and contaminant free.

Conjugated Linoleic Acid (CLA)

CLA is another essential fatty acid that is clinically proven to help you lose weight. This EFA is found naturally in grass fed (finished) beef. Grass fed beef is not fattened just before going to market. Grains fed to beef change the EFAs in the meat, leading to a far less healthy product.

For best results, take all EFAs with a meal.

8. Take a Vitamin/Mineral Supplement

Always take vitamins and minerals with a meal. A supplement in capsule form will digest better than one in tablet form. It is a good idea to take a daily multivitamin and multi-mineral.

Evaluate what is in your supplements; binders, fillers, artificial flavors, artificial colors, and sweeteners are not recommended.

The Get Lean and Healthy system is very effective when implemented with no supplements at all. This is because you're eating large quantities of high quality food loaded with vitamins, minerals, and antioxidants. Don't spend too much money on supplements; instead, save your money for more high quality food. Organic is best.

People lost weight and stayed healthy through diet and exercise long before supplements came into existence. What's needed for health and weight loss is not more supplements, but higher quality foods. High quality foods support the body's requirements.

Stay away from garbage supplements, such as "fat burners" and "carbohydrate blockers." They are a waste of money, are ineffective, and take the emphasis off proper eating.

9. Eat Organic

Certified organic foods are not genetically modified organisms (GMO) and are grown without pesticides. Many regular fruits and vegetables get sprayed up to ten times with toxic pesticides during their growth. Pesticides are toxic. If they were not toxic, they wouldn't be effective for the farmers. They have to be toxic enough to either kill pests or contaminate the food so pests won't eat it. Either way, we ingest toxins.

Organic farmers inevitably lose a very small percentage of their crop, more than regular farmers, leading to slightly higher costs. Less produce is damaged then you might think, however.

10. Eat Wild Fish, Avoid Farmed Fish

All fish is somewhat contaminated with mercury and other toxins.

At the time of writing this book, it's commonly suggested that you limit eating large fish like salmon and tuna. These fish are high on the food chain and, therefore, are more contaminated. Smaller fish like herring and sardines can be eaten more often. By the time you begin reading this book, who knows, it may even be suggested that you eat no fish at all. One thing we can agree on is that all farmed fish are more contaminated than wild fish.

Current consumption suggestions at the time of printing:

Large Farmed Fish	6 times per year
Large Wild Fish	2 times per month
Small Wild Fish	4 times per month

11. Eat less Soy Products

Soy products have three major problem ingredients. The three problem substances in soy are protease inhibitors, phytic acid, and phytoestrogens.

a) Protease Inhibitors

Protease Inhibitors impair the body's ability to digest protein.

b) Phytic Acid (Phytates)

Phytic acid impairs the body's ability to absorb essential mineral such as calcium and zinc.

c) Phytoestrogens

Phytoestrogens are estrogen-like compounds in plants. Estrogen-like compounds in soy have effects like herbs or drugs. For people with certain conditions, phytoestrogens makes sense; for others, they don't. A full explanation of phytoestrogens is outside the scope of this weight loss book, but, for now, just know that soy should be treated a bit like a drug. Limit exposure to soy products to two meals per week or less, unless recommended by your healthcare provider.

12. Only Eat Sprouted Grains and Legumes

Grains and Legumes

Beans (legumes) and grains contain anti-nutrients called phytic acids. Phytic acid (phytates) bind to minerals. Eating too much phytic acid can deplete minerals. Beans are not often promoted in GLH because of their ability to deplete minerals. Legumes are also too high in starch for someone who wants rapid weight loss. Beans can be eaten two to three times per week on the maintenance system, more often if the bean has sprouted.

Ancient people somehow knew about the detrimental effects of phytic acid, so they soaked, fermented, and sprouted their legumes before eating them. Soaking beans for several hours (6-12 hours) before cooking, rinsing them, and cooking in fresh water can reduce phytic acid. Fermenting does a better job of reducing the phytic acid. And sprouting can remove all of the phytic acid. As beans sprout, they become more of a fibrous vegetable than a legume. Sprouted beans are fit for any phase of the GLH.

Reducing Phytic Acid

Good	Soaking (6-12hours)
Better	Fermenting
Best	Sprouting

13. Consume Protein at Every Meal

Consuming high quality protein at every meal will help you lose weight. Protein also gives you steady blood sugar levels and consistent energy. Research shows that just eating more protein can increase glucagon secretions, and reduces the total amount of food eaten at that meal and the next. Good protein sources can be found in the Rapid Weight Loss and Nutrition Basics chapters.

14.   Consume less Alcohol

Alcohol will stop you from losing weight rapidly and it may stop you from losing weight at all.   It has too many calories and too few vitamins, minerals, and antioxidants to have any nutritional value.

Alcoholic beverages and calories:

Beverage:	Calories:
12oz beer	140-150
12oz light beer	100-120
6oz Wine	110-130
1.5oz shot of liquor	100-150
Rum and cola	240
Vodka and cranberry	250
Martini	400

Do not drink alcohol if you have hopes of losing weight quickly.   Drink moderately if you plan to stay lean.

15. Avoid Artificial Sweeteners

Avoid artificial sweeteners which condition the body to continually crave sweet foods.   Natural foods, like pears and strawberries, are sweet, but not as sweet as the refined sugar-filled foods that make the body gain weight. Food and drinks such as candy and colas condition our bodies to want fattening, high in sugar types of foods. To stay lean for life, you simply must get your body used to the taste of real food.   When grapes start tasting sweet, when almond butter spread on an apple tastes like candy, and when plain yogurt does not taste sour anymore, this is when you have conditioned your body to like real food again.   This natural food will keep us lean, healthy, and full of vitality.

Artificial sweeteners have been shown to cause some detrimental side effects in some studies.   Most of the side effects were minor, such as gastric upset or headaches. Some, however, were major, including epilepsy/seizures, depression, brain tumors, autoimmune diseases, shrunken thymus gland, enlarged liver and kidneys, atrophy of the lymph follicles in the spleen and thymus, a reduced growth rate, and a decrease in the red blood cell count.

Most studies showed artificial sweeteners were not unhealthy, if consumed in moderation, but I will err on the side of caution as there have been very few long term studies. I'll stick to eating real food and so should you.

16. Eliminate Preservatives

Preservatives:

Preservatives are toxins added to food to prevent microbes (bacteria, fungus, mold, and etc.) from living in the food. The food needs only to be toxic enough to slow the growth of fungus and bacteria. This is a good thing, because food contaminated with bacteria or mould is not good. However, I feel adding toxins to food, in the form of preservatives, is just as bad. Preservatives found in deli meats have been shown, in some studies, to cause cancer.

The choice to avoid or consume preservatives is up to you. Some preservatives, such as those on fresh fruit, are not disclosed, so you cannot always avoid them.

Clearly, some preservatives are much more harmful than others.

Mild preservatives like sorbic acid and potassium sorbate may act as mild irritants.

Preservatives such as benzoic acid and calcium sulphite are harmful if swallowed, may irritate the eyes and lungs, and may cause skin irritation

Laboratory experiments suggest that sodium nitrite, dimethyl dicarbonate and potassium nitrite, may act as carcinogens (cancer causing substances). They may also cause reproductive disorders. Nitrites should not be a part of your new, healthy lifestyle.

In general don't eat anything with an ingredient you don't know or can't pronounce.

17. Eat more Raw Food

Raw food should be eaten daily. Almost every meal or snack should contain at least some raw fruits or vegetables. Cooked foods have denatured (destroyed or inactive) enzymes. Raw foods are your only food-source for enzymes. The cooking process can also damage fragile vitamins and other food elements. Most people don't eat enough raw foods and raw foods are far superior in terms of their nutritional value.

(Please note, some food elements are actually released by the cooking process, so it is good to have both cooked and raw foods.)

18. Eat more Whole Foods

To eat whole foods means to eat foods not processed or refined in any way. Recommending whole foods may sound a bit like you should eat the peel of your banana, but it's not that. Oh, and don't eat a whole turkey, either. To recommend the consumption of whole foods in this context means unrefined foods. Whole foods have all of the vitamins, minerals, and goodness nature intended.

Instead of eating an apple muffin, eat an apple. Instead of having white bread, eat whole grain bread. Better yet, just have the unrefined grain by itself, eat oatmeal.

Any food containing or comprised of refined sugar, flour, or artificial ingredients is not a whole food. If anything was added or taken away, it's no longer a whole food. For high energy and optimal health, you should only consume whole foods.

19. Eat more Fiber

Fiber will help you lose weight by slowing the rise in blood sugar from a meal. This allows glucagon concentrations to stay high and insulin concentrations to stay moderate, leading to a fit, lean body. Fiber is also good for the health of your colon. Fiber has a cleansing effect on the whole digestive system. Soluble fiber can lower cholesterol levels.

20. Avoid Trans-fats

Trans-fat, and hydrogenated oils, should be avoided. These engineered fats can cause heart disease and adversely affect most systems in the body. They are ten times more dangerous than saturated fat. Experts agree that there is no safe level of consumption. Trans-fats may likely be banned in most countries by the time you read this. Unfortunately, most processed food marketed to children contain trans-fats. Fortunately, most food manufacturers are already removing these dangerous oils from their foods.

How do you know if a food contains trans-fats? Look on the label and record the total fat as well as the three listed types of natural fat. Add up the natural fats and subtract that total from the total fat. The remaining balance are trans-fats.

Example:

A. Add up the natural fats:

Saturated fat	3.2grams
Monounsaturated fat	1.2grams
Polyunsaturated fat	0.8grams
Total natural fat	5.2grams

B. Subtract the natural fat from the total fat:

Total Fat	6.0grams
Total natural fat	5.2grams
Trans-fats	0.8grams

C. The balance is trans-fats:

There are some cases where this won't work. Milk and beef contain a small amount of a natural trans-fat called conjugated linoleic acid (CLA). CLA is safe and is sold as a weight loss supplement; however, fish oil is a better essential fatty acid for weight loss and overall health.

Avoid all consumption of unnatural trans-fats.

21. Avoid Low Fat and Low Carbohydrate Foods

Every cell in your body is surrounded by an important membrane made of fat. If you don't get enough high quality fat, then your body won't be able to replace those old fat molecules as they get worn out. Your brain and nerves are about 80% fat (1/3 polyunsaturated DHA mostly). You need to eat high quality fat on a regular basis to stay healthy.

A low fat food can also mean high sugar. A high sugar diet makes you carry a lot of body-fat due to high insulin levels. A few years ago, they were selling licorice as a healthy fat-free snack. It is fat-free, but as we have pointed out, high sugar consumption also contributes to making you fat.

An item of food that is labeled as "low carb" means the food will likely contain artificial sweeteners. And, as we have already discussed, artificial sweeteners do not contribute to good health. The artificial sweeteners will also keep you craving sweet foods, which is something the GLH system goes against. Eventually, eating these foods on a regular basis will make you gain weight.

Eat real food such as apples, peaches, chicken, eggs, squash, broccoli, red peppers, and blueberries. Natural foods like these will help to keep you healthy and **lean.**

22. Eat More Antioxidant Rich Foods

Antioxidants can literally stop the body from breaking down by oxidation. To see an example of oxidation, try the following example. Cut an apple in half. Leave it on the counter for a few hours. When you come back, it will be brown and mushy. Oxygen in the air has broken down the inside of the apple from oxidation. The inside of the apple contains very little antioxidants, so it oxidizes. It was antioxidants in the skin of the apple which kept it fresh. If you want to stop the apple from going brown, just squeeze some lemon juice on it. Lemon juice has antioxidants that protect the apple; keeping it fresh for a longer period of time. Many people have used lemon juice to keep apples from browning, but most probably didn't know it was the antioxidants in the lemon juice protecting the apple from the process of oxidation.

If you want to slow some of the effects of aging (oxidation), eat more of the foods listed below -- foods with high antioxidant levels. Many other foods also contain lesser amounts of these antioxidants, but for simplification, we've only included those most effective for these purposes.

Vitamin A
The best sources of vitamin A are Cod liver oil, egg yolks, and milk products that contain fat such as whole milk, cream, and butter.

Beta-carotene
Beta-carotene is found in carrots, cantaloupe, pumpkin, squash, sweet potatoes, orange colored vegetables, fruits, and leafy green vegetables.

Lutein
Lutein is found in green leafy green vegetables such as spinach, kale, chard, and collard greens.

Lycopene
Lycopene is found in tomatoes, watermelon, guava, papaya, apricots, and pink grapefruit

Selenium
Selenium is found in Brazil nuts, whole grains, wheat germ, butter, lamb, and fish.

Vitamin C
Citrus fruits, broccoli, kiwi fruit, brussels sprouts, bananas, blueberries, cauliflower, and bell peppers all contain vitamin C.

Vitamin E

Vitamin E is found in almonds, cashews, Brazil nuts, walnuts, pecans, peanuts, wheat germ, cold pressed vegetable oils, sweet potatoes, and mangos.

23. Make Healthy Choices when Eating Out

Dining out is where most people stray from the program. Any decent restaurant will allow you to order your meal without starch and double the vegetables with your protein. You must have and use willpower to order the right foods. This is the only way to lose weight and keep it off. Skip the appetizer and dessert.

24. Exercise More

Below are the three best forms of exercise to get you active and stay lean.

1. Lactic acid producing weight training/resistance training

A burning sensation in the working muscles during weight training lets you know the training will help you burn fat. Sets of 10 to 20 repetitions will elicit this response. Surprisingly, weight training is more beneficial than cardiovascular exercise for weight loss. This is because resistance training can increase your metabolic rate for much longer, leading to days of extra fat melting. Lactic acid weight training also increases the body's production of growth hormone. Growth hormone in adults doesn't actually make you grow, it makes you get leaner. Growth hormone helps you burn fat!

2. Cardiovascular interval training

This is cardiovascular training with alternating periods of high intensity and periods of active rest. An example would be wind-sprints. Sprint the length of the field (high intensity) and walk briskly back to the start line (active rest). Repeat.

3. Any exercise you enjoy

Do exercise you enjoy. Only exercises that you actually do will help you lose weight. Whether dancing, walking, aerobics, yoga, pilates, jogging, pick up games of basketball, or whatever it is that you like to do – do it!

25. Avoid Liquid Sugar – Juice and Cola

Drinking juice and/or cola will make you fat. These popular drinks are high in sugar and are void of our three friends: protein, fat, and fiber. This makes cola and juice fit into the category of fat-gain foods. Imagine a person who drinks two cans of (regular – not diet) pop a day. If he or she quit drinking those 2 soft-drinks and drank water instead, keeping all other variables equal, the person would lose about 25 pounds over the course of a year.

Does it taste so good that you're willing to carry 25 extra pounds, the size of a small child, just to have it?

26. Eat More Super-foods

10 Super-Foods That You Should Eat More Often:

1. Green Vegetables
2. Brightly Colored Vegetables
3. Whole Organic Eggs or Omega 3 Eggs
4. Plain Organic Yogurt
5. Organic Berries
6. Almonds
7. Fish Oil
8. Organic Meats
9. Grass Fed (Finished) Beef
10. Whole High-Fiber Fruits

27. Eat More Yogurt

Quality natural yogurt contains strains of beneficial bacteria which is excellent for digestive system health. Eat yogurt 5-7 times a week or supplement with acidophilus. Acidophilus is the main strain of healthy bacteria found in yogurt.

28. Eat More Omega 3 Eggs

Omega three eggs are an excellent food for keeping you lean and healthy. They contain minerals, vitamins, antioxidants, EFA's, and high quality protein. They are also relatively inexpensive and easy to cook. Eat more eggs.

29. Practice a Daily 12 Hour Liver Fast

The liver detoxifies your blood 24 hours a day. The liver also processes all the food coming into your body. To give the liver a rest, don't eat for 12 hours everyday. If your last meal of the day is at 6:00p.m., don't eat until 6:00a.m. Many people do this without realizing what they are doing. However, those who eat late, at 9:00pm, 10:00pm, and 11:00pm, and have breakfast at 7:00am are not giving their liver much of a rest. The daily twelve hour fast will increase your health – not to mention that stopping those late night feedings will also help you lose weight.

30. Be Aware of What You're Eating

You must be aware and be critical of what you are eating; examine every meal, everyday. This awareness is very important during the weight loss phase and even more so during the maintenance phase.

This doesn't mean you won't make poor choices and eat unhealthy food; we all do. It does mean you have to be aware of these poor food choices and make sure it doesn't happen often.

Pay attention. The combination of willpower and awareness is essential to staying lean for life.

Chapter 8: Caloric Breakdown of the GLH system

Below is a caloric breakdown of the Rapid Weight Loss and the Stay Lean phases, for both a 130 pound and 200 pound person. The calorie content for the Rapid Weight Loss Phase is lower than normal, but it is higher than most weight loss diets. This is made possible due to the increase of fat burning hormones triggered by the Get Lean and Healthy system.

Source: The USDA National Nutrient Database

Approximate Rapid Weight Loss Phase Calorie Breakdown for a 130 pound person: *(4oz palm)*

Meal 1	Nutrition shake (with frozen berries)		
	Yogurt 1cup	61	
	Blueberries 1 cup	79	
	Protein powder 30 grams	114	
Snack	1 Medium apple	72	
Meal 2	Chicken Caesar salad	100	
	(125g chicken breast)	206	
	Whole raw red pepper	43	
	½ Raw cucumber	45	
Snack	2 plums	30	
Meal 3	4oz top sirloin steak	260	
	Grilled sliced zucchini (2)	28	
	Large greek salad	155	**Total: 1193**

Approximate Stay Lean Phase Calorie Breakdown for a 130 pound person: *(4oz palm)*

Meal 1	2 Poached eggs	147	
	Whole grain rye toast (1)	68	
	Butter	102	
	Strawberries	168	
Snack	1 Large orange	86	
Meal 2	Chicken leg (125g)	256	
	Salad with oil and vinegar	136	
	Brown rice (100g)	111	
Snack	Handful of raw almonds	82	
	½ OZ (12) almonds		
Meal 3	4oz top sirloin steak	259	
	Sweet potato	89	
	Large greek salad	160	**Total: 1664**

Approximate Rapid Weight Loss Phase Calorie Breakdown for a 200 pound person: *(6oz palm)*

Meal 1	Nutrition shake (with frozen berries)		
	Yogurt 1cup	61	
	Blueberries 1cup	79	
	Protein powder	114	
Snack	1 Large apple	110	
Meal 2	Chicken Caesar salad	100	
	(200g chicken breast)	330	
	Whole raw red pepper	43	
	½ Raw cucumber	45	
Snack	2 plums	30	
Meal 3	6oz top sirloin steak	391	
	Grilled sliced zucchini (3)	42	
	Large greek salad	160	**Total: 1505**

Approximate Stay Lean Phase Calorie Breakdown for a 200 pound person: *(6oz palm)*

Meal 1	4 Poached eggs	294
	Whole grain rye toast (2)	136
	Butter (1 tbsp)	102
	Strawberries (1cup)	168
Snack	1 Large orange	86
Meal 2	2 Chicken legs (200g)	410
	Salad with oil and vinegar	136
	Brown rice (150g)	166
Snack	Handful of raw almonds	164
	1 OZ (23) almonds	
Meal 3	Lamb chops (150g)	300
	Sweet potato (150g)	135
	Large greek salad	160	**Total: 2257**

Chapter 9: Product Comparison

Many foods contain artificial ingredients. These foods are not the way nature intended them to be. The human body was designed to eat whole, unrefined, natural foods. Artificial colors, sweeteners, and preservatives are chemicals the human body has not yet had time to adapt to. Below is a product comparison of similar foods; one with natural ingredients and the other with artificial ingredients. You'll be surprised at how many unnecessary artificial ingredients are in most foods, and you'll soon be surprised at how few ingredients are in quality natural foods.

Start reading ingredient lists. As a rule, if you don't recognize what's in a product, don't eat it.

The ingredients on an ingredient list are written in order from greatest quantity to least. The first ingredient listed is the ingredient in the highest amount. The last ingredient listed is the lowest amount. Sometimes two types of sugar are used, but they will be lower on the ingredient list. If only one type of sugar is used, sugar is the first ingredient. Either way, the product is more sugar than anything else.

In the examples below, the **bold** ingredients are artificial.
The *ITALICIZED CAPITAL* ingredients are types of added sugar.

1a: Turkey (Deli "Oven Roasted")

Ingredients: Turkey, water, *CORN SYRUP SOLIDS*, salt, flavor, egg yolk powder, wheat germ, **sodium nitrate**, *SUGAR*, **caramel color, sodium carbonate.**

1b: Turkey (Roasted in the oven at home by you)

Ingredients: Turkey

Obviously cooking and eating turkey you cooked yourself or that was prepared without sugar and preservatives is better for you. Sodium nitrate, as listed above in 1a, is a carcinogen.

2a: Salsa – Brand 1

Ingredients: Tomatoes in juice, water, onions, tomato paste, peppers (sweet green and jalapeno), salt, lemon juice, white vinegar, dried onion, seasonings, **calcium chloride, citric acid, propionic acid, potassium sorbate.**

2b: Salsa – Brand 2

Ingredients: Tomatoes, water, fresh jalapeno peppers, onions, tomato paste, white vinegar, salt, dehydrated onions, garlic.

Obviously, salsa can be made without preservatives; certainly less than 4 preservatives. (The only downside to food containing fewer preservatives is that it won't last as long in the refrigerator after opening it.)

3a: Peanut Butter – Brand 1

Ingredients: Selected peanuts, corn, *DEXTRIN, SUGAR,* hydrogenated vegetable oil (to prevent separation), salt.

3b: Peanut Butter – Brand 2

Ingredients: Peanuts

Peanut butter should contain only peanuts. Dextrin is sugar. Again, there are two types of sugar in the product listed as 3a. Quite possibly, there is also more total sugar than peanuts in this product. Nut butters (almond, peanut, and cashew) will separate over time, with the oil rising to the top. Just stir to mix in the oil and store in the fridge to prevent separation.

Poor Products, Poor Ingredients

Below are a couple of examples of products to be avoided and why.

Hearty Chicken Soup

Ingredients: Water, chicken broth, carrots, macaroni (enriched wheat flour, egg whites), chicken, celery, chicken fat, salt, potato starch, hydrolyzed plant protein (corn, soy, wheat), **monosodium glutamate**, *SUGAR*, **yeast extract**, onion powder, dehydrated parsley, **flavor**, spice

This soup contains yeast extract, which is actually mono-sodium glutamate (MSG). Note that monosodium gluta-mate (MSG) is listed in the product as well. There is a lot of MSG in this product! It is hard to find prepared soup without artificial ingredients. Carefully read the ingredients of all prepared soups and dinners.

Tomato Ketchup

Ingredients: Tomato paste (made from fresh ripe toma-toes), white vinegar, *LIQUID SUGAR, FRUCTOSE SYRUP,* salt, onion powder, spices

There are two types of sugar in this product. Basically, ketchup is made from tomatoes, sugar, and vinegar. There are no artificial ingredients, because the vinegar acts as a preservative, but ketchup has so much sugar you really need to think of it as candy. Most BBQ sauces should be thought of as candy as well.

Chapter 10: Choose your Body

Decide today that healthy eating and exercise are permanent lifestyle changes you are committed to. Set a higher standard for yourself and refuse to eat unhealthy food. Refuse to eat food that will make you fat. Treat your body like a temple, one that you will want to honor and respect for the remainder of your life. Treat your body as if it's the only one you'll ever get, because it really is. There is no walk away lease on your body. You can't trade it in for a new one, no matter what makeover television programs make us want to believe.

If you ever find yourself putting weight back on, just return to the Rapid Weight Loss phase and quickly shed those excess pounds. Really, this is the simplest diet ever. Three meals of a palm sized protein with an unlimited amount of high fiber vegetables, plus two snacks, one mid-morning and one mid-afternoon, consisting of a fist sized portion of high fiber fruit. The system is simple, healthy, and effective.

Keep this book as a reference. Refer to it often to make sure you stay lean and provide your body with the best nutrition possible.

Remember what you have learned. You cannot be overweight and optimally healthy. If you want to live a longer and healthier life, commit yourself to living the healthy principles in this book. Give your body the best nutrition possible and try to exercise a little each day.

With every meal, you're choosing your body because you really are what you eat. With every workout you do or skip, you're also choosing your body. Every decision regarding food, water, alcohol, and exercise is a decision about what kind of body you will have. Do you want a lean, fit and healthy body? Do you really? If yes, it's within your reach.

I want to personally wish you the best of luck getting the lean and healthy body you deserve. There may be setbacks along the way, but with persistence you will succeed. Decide now how you want things to be. You can do anything you set your mind to and overcome any obstacle you set your sights on. All you need to do is go for it!

Get Lean and Healthy Summary

Here's the program in a nutshell: eat 5-6 times per day, 3 meals and 2-3 snacks. Eat following the template below and follow this program 100% of the time. If you stay consistent, you can expect to lose 4-12 pound the first week and 1-3 pounds every week there after.

Rapid Weight Loss Program Rules:

1. The Palm Rule
Each meal must consist of a palm sized portion of protein eaten with unlimited greens and fibrous vegetables. Eat a fist sized portion of high fiber fruit or a handful of raw almonds as a snack between meals.

2. The Three Hour Rule
Never go more than 3 hours without eating. However, do not eat late; you should go 12 hours from your last meal before having breakfast.

3. The Water Rule
Drink 1L (or just over four cups) of water for every 50 pounds of bodyweight per day. Drink only water, green tea, herbal tea; and black tea; do not drink cola, juice, or sports drinks.

4. The Exercise Rule

Exercise vigorously for at least 30 minutes every day. (If you can't exercise daily, make sure you do about 3-4 hours per week total.)

5. The Natural Food Rule

Whenever possible, eat natural, whole, and preferably organic foods.

Rapid Weight Loss Phase Outline (1000-1500Kcal)

Meal 1   Protein – palm sized portion
Fruit – palm sized portion (no bananas)
Natural/plain yogurt – palm sized portion
or
Nutrition Shake   - 1cup plain yogurt
   - 1cup frozen berries
   - ½ cup water
   - 1 scoop whey protein isolate
   Blend and enjoy

Snack   Fruit – fist sized portion
or
a handful of raw almonds

Meal 2   Protein – palm sized portion
Fibrous vegetables – unlimited

Snack   Fruit – fist sized portion
or
a handful of raw almonds

Meal 3   Protein – palm sized portion
Fibrous vegetables – unlimited

(There are no refined sugar, flour products, starchy vegetables, grains, or legumes consumed in the Rapid Weight Loss phase.)

Plate Templates

Rapid Weight Loss Meal

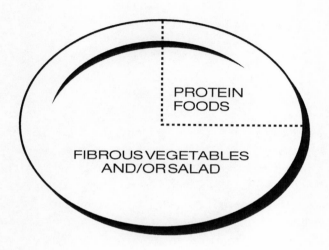

Maintenance Meal

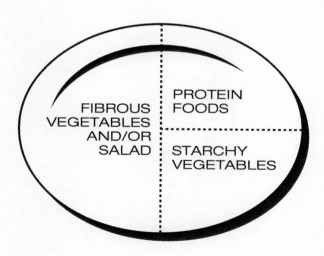

Progress Journal

In this weight loss journal, you should enter in your weekly weight and the date of the weigh-in to keep track of your progress. 52 weeks worth of entries have been included here for your use. If you keep this system up and follow your progress for a full year, you will be well on your way for a lifetime of healthy living. For weeks where you do not lose much weight, or maybe you lost more than expected, add comments from your food journal (an example is provided later in this chapter) to help you remember what happened (did you splurge on a cola or starch, skip snacks, each more/less fruit, exercise more/less, etc.).

Get Lean and Healthy
Weight Loss Journal

Name:

Start Weight:

Start Date:

	Date	Weight	Comments
Week 1			
Week 2			
Week 3			
Week 4			
Week 5			
Week 6			
Week 7			
Week 8			
Week 9			
Week 10			
Week 11			
Week 12			
Week 13			
Week 14			
Week 15			
Week 16			
Week 17			
Week 18			
Week 19			

	Date	Weight	Comments
Week 20			
Week 21			
Week 22			
Week 23			
Week 24			
Week 25			
Week 26			
Week 27			
Week 28			
Week 29			
Week 30			
Week 31			
Week 32			
Week 33			
Week 34			
Week 35			
Week 36			
Week 37			
Week 38			

	Date	Weight	Comments
Week 39			
Week 40			
Week 41			
Week 42			
Week 43			
Week 44			
Week 45			
Week 46			
Week 47			
Week 48			
Week 49			
Week 50			
Week 51			
Week 52			

Start Weight:

End Weight:

First Week Weight Loss:

Eight Week Weight Loss:

Total Weight Lost:

Date:	Monday	Tuesday	Wednesday
Day:	MEAL 1	MEAL 1	MEAL 1
Month:			
Year:	SNACK 1	SNACK 1	SNACK 1
In this food journal, you should list everything you put into your mouth. List all consumed food and beverages, even hard candies and gum.	MEAL 2	MEAL 2	MEAL 2
	SNACK 2	SNACK 2	SNACK 2
	MEAL 3	MEAL 3	MEAL 3
	SNACK 3	SNACK 3	SNACK 3
	WATER	WATER	WATER

www.getleansystem.com

FOOD JOURNAL

Thursday	Friday	Saturday	Sunday
MEAL 1	MEAL 1	MEAL 1	MEAL 1
SNACK 1	SNACK 1	SNACK 1	SNACK 1
MEAL 2	MEAL 2	MEAL 2	MEAL 2
SNACK 2	SNACK 2	SNACK 2	SNACK 2
MEAL 3	MEAL 3	MEAL 3	MEAL 3
SNACK 3	SNACK 3	SNACK 3	SNACK 3
WATER	WATER	WATER	WATER

Resources

Ascherio A, Rimm ER, Giovannucci EL, Colditz GA, Rosner B, Willett WC, Sacks F, Stampfer MJ. A prospective study of nutritional factors and hypertension among US men. Circulation. 1992 Nov; 86(5): 1475-84.

Barkeling B, Rossner S, Bjorvell H. Effects of a high-protein meal (meat) and a high-carbohydrate meal (vegetarian) on satiety measured by automated computerized monitoring of subsequent food intake, motivation to eat and food preferences. Int J Obes 1990; 14:743-751.

Barzel US. The skeleton as an ion exchange system: implications for the role of acid-base imbalance in the genesis of osteoporosis. J Bone Min Res 1995; 10:1431-1436.

Bowen J, et al. A high dietary protein, high-calcium diet minimizes bone turnover in overweight adults during weight loss. J Nutr. 2004 Mar:134(3):568-73.

Burger J, et al. Heavy metals in commercial fish in New Jersey. Environ Res. 2005 Nov;99(3):403-12.

Burger J et al. Mercury in commercial fish; optimizing individual choices to reduce risk. Environ Health Perspect. 2005Mar;113(3):266-71.

Brekke HK, et al. Lifestyle modification improves risk factors inn type 2 diabetes relatives. Diabetes Res Clin Pract. 2005; April68(1);18-28.

Carel RA, et al. Education on the glycemic index of foods fails to improve treatment outcomes in a behavioral weight loss program. Eat Behav. 2005 Feb,^(2):145-50.

Cordain L, Miller JB, Eaton SB, Mann N. Macronutrient estimations in hunter-gatherer diets. Am J Clin Nutr. 2000 Dec;72(6): 1589-92.

Cordain L., Watkins. Increased dietary protein modifies glucose and insulin homeostasis in adult women during weight loss. J. Nutri. Feb;133(2):405-10.

Davidson, et al. Neurodevelopmental outcomes of Seychellois children from the pilot cohort at 108 months following prenatal exposure to methylmercury from a maternal fish diet. Environ Res. 2000 Sep;84(1):1-11.

Davis MS, et al. More favorable dietary patterns are associated with lower glycemic load in older adults. J Am Diet Assoc. 2004 Dec;104(12):1828-35.

Diepvens K, et al. Metabolic effects of green tea and phases of weight loss. Physiol Behav. 2005 Nov.

Dulloo AG, et al. Efficacy of a green tea extract rich in catechin polyphenols and caffeine in increasing 24-h energy expenditure and fat oxidation in humans
Am J Clin Nutr. 1999 Dec;70: 1040 - 1045.

Dyck DJ. Leptin sensitivity in skeletal muscle is modulated by diet and exercise. Exerc Sport Sci Rev. 2005 Oct:33(4);189-194.

Eaton SB, Cordain L. Evolutionary aspects of diet: old genes, new fuels. Nutritional changes since agriculture. World Rev Nutr Diet. 1997;81:26-37.

Ebbeling CB, et al. A reduced-glycemic load diet in the treatment of adolescent obesity. Arch Pediatr Adolesc Med. 2003 Aug;157(8):773-9.

Foster GD, et al. A randomized trial of a low-carbohydrate diet for obesity. N Engl J Med. 2003 May22;348(21):2082-90.

Griffin, Sean & Cuddeford, Vijay, The CancerSmart Consumer Guide. Labour Environmental Alliance Society, April 2004.

Goodpaster BH, et al. Enhanced fat oxidation through physical activity is associated with improvements in insulin sensitivity in obesity. Diabetes. 2003 Sep:52(9);2191-7.

Gumbiner B, et al. Effects of a monounsaturated fatty acid-enriched hypocaloric diet on cardiovascular risk factors in obese patients with type 2 diabetes. Diabetes Care. 1998 Jan;21(1):9-15.

Haas, Elson M. Staying Healthy with Nutrition. Celestial Arts. 1992.

Hurrell, R. Influence of Vegetable Protein Sources on Trace Element and Mineral Bioavailability. The American Society for Nutritional Sciences J. Nutr. 133:2973S-2977S, September 2003.

Jeffery RW, et al. Physical activity and weight loss: does prescribing higher activity goals improve outcome? Am J Clin Nutr. 2003 Oct;78(4):684-9.

Kataria, et al. Antinutrients in amphidilipids (black gram x Mung bean): varietal differences and effects of domestic processing and cooking. Plant Foods Hum Nutr. 1989 Sep;39(3):257-66.

Keaton KW, et al. Not just fibre – the nutritional consequences of refined carbohydrate foods. Hum Nutr Clin Nutr. 1983 Jan:37(1):31-5.

Kille JW, et al. Sucralose: lack of effects on sperm glycolysis and reproduction in the rat. Food Chem Toxicol. 2000;38 Suppl 2:S19-29.

Labayen I, et al. Effects of protein vs. carbohydrate-rich diets on fuel utilization in obsess women during weight loss. Forum Nutr. 2003;56;168-70.

Lau K, et al. Synergistic Interactions Between Commonly Used Food Additives in a Developmental Neurotoxicity Test. Toxicol Sci. 2005 Dec 13.

Layman DK, et al. Plasma leptin concentrations in Pima Indians living in drastically different environments. Diabetes care. 1999 Mar;22(3):413-7.

Leslie WS, Lean ME, Baillie HM, Hankey CR. Weight management: a comparison of existing dietary approaches in a work-site setting. Int J Obes Relat Metab Disord. 2002 Nov, 26(11):1469-75.

Liu S, et al. A prospective study of dietary glycemic load, carbohydrate intake, and risk of coronary heart disease in US women. Am J Clin Nutr. 2000 Jun; 71(6);1455-61.

Lofgren I, et al. Weigh loss associated with reduced intake of carbohydrate reduces the atherogenicity of LDL in premenopausal women. Metabolism. 2005 Sep;54(9):1133-41.

Lombardo YB, Chicco AG. Effects of polyunsaturated n-3 fatty acids on dyslipidemia and insulin resistance in rodents and in humans. A review. J Nutr Biochem. 2006 Jan; 17(1):1-13.

Lucchini R, et al. Neurotoxic effect of exposure to low doses of mercury. Med Lav. 2002 May-June;93 (3):202-14. Italian.

Ludwig DS, et al. High glycemic index foods, overeating and obesity. Pediatrics. 1999 Mar;103(3):E26.

Luscombe-Marsh ND, et al. Carbohydrate restricted diets high in either monounsaturated fat or protein are equally effective at promoting fat loss and improving blood lipids. Am J Nutr. 2005 Apr;8(4):762-72.

Marianne BM van den Bree, et al. Genetic and environmental influences on eating patterns of twins aged 50 y. Am. J. Clin Nutr, 1999 Oct; 70: 456 - 465.

Melanson K, et al. Weight loss and total lipid profile changes in overweight women consuming beef or chicken as the primary protein source. Nutrition. 2003 May;19(5):409-14.

Nelson GJ, et al. Low–fat diets do not lower plasma cholesterol levels in healthy men compared to high-fat diets with similar fatty acid composition at constant caloric intake. Lipids. Nov; 30(11); 969-76.

Oh R. Practical applications of fish oil (Omega3 fatty acids) in primary care. J Am Board Fam Pract. 2005 Jan-Feb;18(1):28-36.

Olney JW. Excitotoxins in foods.
Neurotoxicology. 1994 Fall;15(3):535-44.

Olney JW. Excitotoxic food additives--relevance of animal studies to human safety.
Neurobehav Toxicol Teratol. 1984 Nov-Dec;6(6):455-62.

Parker B, et al. Effect of high-protein, high monounsaturated fat weight loss diet on glycemic control and lipid levels in type 2 diabetes. Diabetes Care. 2002 Mar;25(3):425-30.

Piatti PM, et al. Hypocaloric high-protein diet improves glucose oxidation and spares lean body mass: comparison to hypocaloric high-carbohydrate diet. Metabolism. 1994 Dec;43(12):1481-7.

Reddy MB, et al. The impact of food processing on nutritional quality of vitamins and minerals. Adv Exp Med Biol. 1999;459:99-106.

Rossi AS, et al. Dietary fish oil positively regulated plasma leptin levels and adiponectin levels in sucrose-fed, insulin resistance rats. Am J Physiol Regu Integr Comp Physiol. 2005 Aug;289(2):R486-R494.

Ruzickova J, et al. Omega-# PUFA of marine origin limit diet-induced obesity in mice by reducing cellularity of adipose tissue. Lipids. 2004 Dec;39(12):1177-85.

Saharan k, et al. Processing of newly released ricebean and fababean cultivars: changes in total and available calcium, iron and phosphorus. Int J Food Sci Nutr. 2001 Sep;52(5):413-8.

Sasaki YF, et al.The comet assay with 8 mouse organs: results with 39 currently used food additives. Mutat Res. 2002 Aug 26;519(1-2):103-19.

Schulze MB, et al. Glycemic index, glycemic load, and dietary fiber intake and incidence of type @ diabetes in younger and middle-aged women. Am J Clin Nutr. 2004 Aug;80(2):348-56.

Simopoulos AP, et al. Omega-3 fatty acids in health and disease and in growth and development. Am J Clin Nutr. 1991 Sep;54(3) 438-63. Review.

Smith JD, et al. Relief of fibromyalgia symptoms following discontinuation of dietary excitotoxins. Ann Pharmacother. 2001 Jun;35(6):702-6.

Somers V, et al. Fish-rich tribal diet linked with low leptin levels. Rapid Access Issue, Circulation. July 2, 2002.

Wallace AM, et al. Plasma leptin and the risk of cardiovascular disease in the west of Scotland coronary prevention study (WOSCOPS). Circulation 2001 Dec 18;104(25):3052-6.

Warren JM, et al. Low glycemic index breakfasts and reduced food intake in preadolescent children. Pediatrics. 2003 Nov;112(5):e414.

Weigle DS, et al. A high-protein diet induces sustained reductions in appetite, ad libitum caloric intake, and body weight despite compensatory changes in diurnal plasma leptin and ghrelin concentrations. Am J Clin Nutr. 2005 Jul;82(1):41-8.

Wolever TM, Bolognesi C. Prediction of glucose and insulin responses of normal subjects after consuming mixed meals varying in energy, protein, fat carbohydrate and glycemic index. J Nutr 1996;126: 2807-2812.

Wolever TM, Relationship between dietary fiber content and composition in foods and the glycemic index. Am J Clin Nutr. 1990 Jan;5(1):72-5.

Wolever TM, et al. Second-meal effect: low glycemic-index foods eaten at dinner improve subsequent breakfast glycemic response. AM J CLin Nutr. 1988 Oct;48(4):1041-7.

Yokoo EM, et al. Low level methylmercury exposure effects neuropsychological function in adults. Environ Health. 2003 Jun 4;2(1):8.

Online Resources

http://www.chm.bris.ac.uk/webprojects2001/anderson/preservatives.htm
http://www.mercola.com/
http://www.westonaprice.org/
http://www.nal.usda.gov/fnic/foodcomp/search/

About the Author

With more than ten years of experience, Todd Matthews is dedicated to the field of health and human performance. He services a diverse spectrum of clients, from high level athletes to once sedentary individuals, ranging in age from 14 to 84. His specialty is getting ordinary people into extraordinary shape through exercise and nutrition.

His experience combined with an extensive educational background make Todd Matthews an expert in his field. He holds a degree from Ryerson University, a diploma in Natural Nutrition, and is an NSCA Certified Strength and Conditioning Specialist. As a Registered Holistic Nutritionist and RNCP, Todd works with his clients to achieve healthy weight loss and increased athletic performance.